T0221750

Antivaccination and Vaccine Hesitancy

This important book provides a comprehensive guide to understanding vaccine hesitancy, as well as the nuances of antivaccination claims. It is designed to give clinicians and other professionals targeted information to help them address vaccine hesitancy and antivaccination claims, as well as ways of responding to immunisation concerns.

Alongside the scientific facts around vaccinations, it considers the historical foundations of modern vaccine scepticism, while offering key insights into the psychology behind vaccine hesitancy and the factors which influence an individual's decision-making. Separating fact from fiction, the book explores the most well-known antivaccine myths, many of which proliferate online, uncovering ways that counter-vaccine narratives can influence audiences. Importantly, it also outlines the most effective strategies to address both doubts and misinformation, detailing five general principles to improve communications, with tips and guidance to debunk false claims or provide assurance in the face of immunisation doubts.

This is essential reading for anyone wishing to really understand the phenomenon of vaccine hesitancy, whether professional, student or general reader, and the methods that can be used to challenge misinformation.

Thomas Aechtner is an Associate Professor in the Faculty of Humanities and Social Sciences at the University of Queensland. As a Westpac Research Fellow alumnus, and a recipient of UQ's Foundation Research Excellence Award, his research examines vaccine hesitancy, antievolutionism, religion-science conflict, media persuasion, and public perceptions of science. He holds a doctorate from the University of Oxford, an MA from the University of Calgary, and a BSc in Biological Sciences from the University of Alberta.

Antivaccination and Vaccine Hesitancy

A Professional Guide to Foster Trust and Tackle Misinformation

Thomas Aechtner

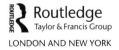

Routledge
Taylor & Francis Group

LONDON AND NEW YORK

Designed cover image: © Getty Images

First published 2024
by Routledge
4 Park Square, Milton Park, Abingdon, Oxon OX14 4RN

and by Routledge
605 Third Avenue, New York, NY 10158

Routledge is an imprint of the Taylor & Francis Group, an informa business

© 2024 Thomas Aechtner

British Library Cataloguing-in-Publication Data
A catalogue record for this book is available from the British Library

Library of Congress Cataloging-in-Publication Data
Names: Aechtner, Thomas, author.
Title: Antivaccination and vaccine hesitancy : a professional guide to foster trust and tackle misinformation / Thomas Aechtner.
Description: Milton Park, Abingdon, Oxon ; New York, NY : Routledge, 2024. | Includes bibliographical references and index.
Identifiers: LCCN 2023009456 (print) | LCCN 2023009457 (ebook) | ISBN 9781032320519 (hardback) | ISBN 9781032320496 (paperback) | ISBN 9781003312550 (ebook)
Subjects: LCSH: Vaccine hesitancy. | Anti-vaccination movement.
Classification: LCC RA638 .A39 2024 (print) | LCC RA638 (ebook) | DDC 614.4--dc23/eng/20230527
LC record available at https://lccn.loc.gov/2023009456
LC ebook record available at https://lccn.loc.gov/2023009457

ISBN: 978-1-032-32051-9 (hbk)
ISBN: 978-1-032-32049-6 (pbk)
ISBN: 978-1-003-31255-0 (ebk)

DOI: 10.4324/9781003312550

Typeset in Bembo
by Taylor & Francis Books

To Ben and Xander

Contents

Illustrations

Figures

Table

Acknowledgements

This book is a product of a Westpac Research Fellowship, funded by the Westpac Scholars Trust. I am indebted to the trust's generous support over the years, and its willingness to back research into vaccine hesitancy. This book would also not exist without the dedicated help of the University of Queensland's Institute for Teaching and Learning Innovation's UQx team. I am particularly grateful to Samantha Briggs, Shannon O'Brien, Anne-Maree Jaggs, and Catherine Coogan West. This brilliant group of people delivered unwavering assistance in producing AVAXX101, the edX course from which this book evolved. I further acknowledge support received through the University of Queensland's Foundation Research Excellence Award. Key findings resulting from UQFREA funded research is featured within this book's chapters.

The greatest debt, however, is owed to my wife Mindy. She has supported my academic pursuits from their earliest beginnings, accompanying me from Canada to England, and then to Australia where we are now fortunate to live. I am, as always, extraordinarily thankful to be married to her, my beloved. I am also grateful to be able to help raise our boys Ben and Xander with her. Being their father is one of life's ultimate privileges.

Abbreviations

DCD	Distrust, Confidence, and Danger
DTP	Diphtheria, tetanus, pertussis
ELM	Elaboration Likelihood Model
Hib	Haemophilus Influenzae Type B
HPV	Human Papillomavirus
ITP	Idiopathic thrombocytopenic purpura
MI	Motivational Interviewing
MMR	Measles, mumps, rubella
OARS	Open-ended questions, Affirmation, Reflecting, and Summary
OPV	Oral polio vaccine

1 Understanding vaccination and antivaccination

In 2021, when COVID-19 vaccine rollouts were launching across the world, several people began to confide in me about their vaccination fears. Colleagues, friends, and strangers related stories about dangers they had heard about. Some expressed how it seemed as though the new vaccines were improperly tested and rushed into production. I received texts from acquaintances, explaining that they had been told getting vaccinated with the "experimental" COVID-19 vaccines would lead to infertility. A fellow researcher at my university whispered unease to me about the risks of vaccine-related blood clots. In coming months, another colleague stormed out of a meeting, enraged that newly introduced work mandates would require her to be vaccinated. Necessitating vaccines, she insisted, was undemocratic. When I went to get my haircut, the hairdresser asked whether I had heard the latest news about mRNA vaccines? They were incredibly unsafe, she confided, because they could alter our DNA. I also received several emails from members of the public, which accused the Government, as well as myself, of colluding with BigPharma for malicious ends. As the pandemic continued a relative of mine announced that every person under the age of 50 who had received a COVID-19 vaccine would drop dead within the next five years.

Each of these encounters related to vaccines in the SARS-CoV-2 pandemic. However, they were also representative of a wider range of arguments and anxieties about vaccines that have been voiced long before the age of COVID-19. In fact, worries about possible vaccine risks, as well as vocal opposition to mandatory vaccination policies, have existed for almost as long as vaccines have. Additionally, early apprehensions about vaccines, and past grievances against compulsory vaccination acts, frequently parallel the types of assertions made about vaccines and immunisation policies in the present day. The claims and fears that people have aired about vaccines throughout history are surprisingly similar to modern vaccination worries. These commonalities are important, because they embody core disputes and doubts about vaccines that continue to have real world consequences, including outbreaks of preventable diseases. This is why in 2019 the World Health Organization listed vaccine hesitancy as one of the top ten global

DOI: 10.4324/9781003312550-1

health threats.[1] During this same year, before COVID-19 made vaccines a daily frontpage news topic, I also proposed that my employer, the University of Queensland, should host a free online course dedicated to addressing antivaccination and vaccine hesitancy.[2] My research involves examining science scepticism, including antivaccination persuasion, vaccine hesitancy, antievolutionism, public perceptions of science, and mass media. In studying these topics, a persistent theme emerged: though academics have continued to identify what seems to lie behind science scepticism, there can be lack of easily accessible, comprehensive training on science scepticism, antivaccination and vaccine hesitancy.[3] With the help of my university's Institute for Teaching and Learning Innovation, I set out to help tackle that deficit. This book is one of the products of that reckless venture. Its goal is to untangle vaccine hesitancy and antivaccination claims, while also mapping out optimal ways of responding to immunisation concerns.

This volume features central insights into the psychological tendencies that lie behind why people have vaccine worries. It also reveals what sociocultural factors influence vaccine decision-making, while covering the science and safety of vaccines. This includes exploring many of the most widespread antivaccine myths and persuasion strategies. In doing so, this book not only provides genuine vaccination facts, but it also uncovers the striking ways that counter-vaccine narratives continue to influence audiences around the world. Importantly, upcoming chapters outline the most effective strategies identified for addressing vaccine doubts expressed by hesitant patients, friends, or relatives. This includes five general principles for improving pro-vaccine communications, and tips for more effectively debunking misinformation. Altogether, it offers a suite of practical advice about vaccine refusal, and research-based methods that can be implemented to improve vaccine advocacy. Before diving into these topics, however, it is necessary to examine what the terms antivaccination and vaccine hesitancy actually refer to. This reveals that they are not necessarily one and the same thing.

What is vaccine hesitancy?

For countless people vaccinations are simply part of the mundane routines of life. Vast numbers of individuals were vaccinated during childhood, and if they went on to have their own kids, they got them vaccinated as recommended by their family physicians. For many, flu shots are an annual custom, and when traveling abroad people ensure that they are up to date with the vaccines needed to keep themselves protected from disease. This commonplace nature of vaccines may cause the general public to overlook the colossal impacts of vaccination on global health. Despite seeming to be a banal part of our lives, vaccines represent one of the most effective medical breakthroughs in human history, and save millions of lives every year.[4] Nevertheless, despite the clear health outcomes of vaccines, opposition to vaccination has existed for over a century. The first references to "anti-vaccinators" appear at the very start of the 19th century, and the percentage of books which contain the words "anti-vaccination" or "antivaccination" spiked in the decades following the introduction of the first state-sponsored vaccination campaigns.[5] By the end of the 20th century, however, references to antivaccination had dropped dramatically, before they once again started rising sharply from the 1990s to the present-day. That rise has continued, and there remained a growing interest and concern over antivaccination from the end of the 20th century, into the 21st.

The terms *antivaccination* and *antivaccinationist* usually refer to vocal, ardent vaccine denial, and a refusal to be vaccinated, designating the active rejection of scientific consensus on vaccines. What is important about these categories is that while they may apply to a particular segment of any given society, the percentage of people who might be classified as antivaccinationist tend to represent relatively smaller shares of the public in most countries.[6] Apart from that, avid vaccine denial and refusal does not suitably describe a broad spectrum of people who might simply have questions or worries about vaccines. Maintaining concerns about what ingredients are in vaccines, or reservations about how many vaccines a child should receive at any one time, does not necessarily make someone an antivaccinationist. The term, antivaccination can also be quite polarising, and an oversimplification that may involve characterising people as either antivaccinationist on one hand, or fully supportive of vaccines on the other. As it turns out, there is a lot of middle ground between those two polar options.[7]

This middle ground includes people who have received all their recommended vaccinations, who have had their family members vaccinated, yet who still express some doubts about the safety and effectiveness of vaccines. It can also be made up of individuals who might accept some but not all vaccines, as well as people who choose to delay certain vaccines for their children. Consequently, a continuum of views exists between those members of the population who accept vaccines without uncertainties, and those who totally refuse all vaccines (Figure 1.1). This spectrum is comprised of individuals who choose to get vaccinated but still have misgivings, as well as others who may refuse some but not all vaccines, or those who delay

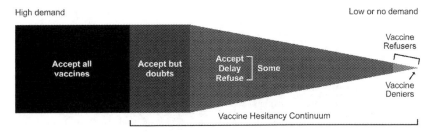

Figure 1.1 The Vaccine Hesitancy Continuum[9]

vaccination and fail to keep their children up to date with all of the recommended immunisations. In recognising that populations reveal such complexities that extend beyond unswerving antivaccination and resolute vaccine acceptance, researchers have developed the term *vaccine hesitancy* to depolarize matters.[8]

Vaccine hesitancy refers to assorted reasons why someone might question, delay, or refuse vaccinations in the context of a decision-making process around vaccination.[10] The term includes varying degrees of concern about vaccines, their safety, and doubts about their necessity, as well as a range of behaviours taken in response to such concerns. The scope of vaccine hesitancy, therefore, includes everyone who is not classified as a wholehearted vaccine acceptor; from those who accept vaccines but still have doubts, to ardent vaccine deniers. This means that vaccine hesitancy is broader and more complex than the term antivaccination. Plus, the number of people who express vaccine hesitancy includes a far larger percentage of the population than only those who might be classified as committed vaccine rejectors.

The extensive scope of vaccine hesitancy makes it challenging to draw a general picture of individuals who express it. This is because people who have anxieties and questions about vaccination can come from a variety of backgrounds, and they can convey distinct hesitations for different vaccines. For instance, some might feel thoroughly comfortable with the Hepatitis B vaccine, but have qualms about the measles, mumps, and rubella shot, or be particularly uncomfortable with newer vaccines, such as those developed to prevent COVID-19. As things stand, vaccine hesitancy has proven to be particularly complicated, and people's vaccination worries can be shaped by a wide variety of factors. These include whether people trust in the safety of vaccines, or if individuals have confidence in the medical system and healthcare professionals. Vaccine hesitancy can be sparked by a lack of trust in pharmaceutical companies and governments, or whether people have had positive experiences discussing vaccines with their local family physician in the past. Social ties and cultural beliefs, shared with an individual's family, friends and community networks, can also predispose some to resist vaccines. Added to all these factors may also be political and media influences, which can impact people's vaccination decisions. As a result, there is often no single source of vaccine hesitancy. Plus, because vaccine hesitancy is featured across a spectrum of attitudes and behaviours, people with vaccination uncertainties cannot simply be pigeonholed into one clear-cut group or characterisation.

This complexity is both the key, and the challenge, of vaccine hesitancy. While only a comparatively small fraction of the population may be genuinely antivaccinationist, a much larger proportion of people convey vaccine hesitancy. Such individuals represent different backgrounds, beliefs, and life experiences that can fuel doubts about the necessity and safety of vaccines. This may include you, if you have ever had some misgivings about certain vaccines, or your friends and family, who might have shared rumours about potential vaccination risks similar to those that I was told about COVID-19 vaccines. Crucially, the sheer breadth and intricacy of vaccine hesitancy is also why it is necessary to look beyond the very narrow term antivaccination. This is because when it comes to public confidence in immunisation, and the importance of maintaining sufficient vaccination rates to avoid preventable disease outbreaks, we need to consider the potentially much greater numbers of people who are not necessarily antivaccine, but who may *still* harbour vaccine hesitancy. With that in mind, it is also essential to consider further questions connected to the dilemma of vaccine hesitancy, including: Why do people have such uncertainties in the first place, and what can be done to better address these doubts in order to keep vaccination coverage high? Before trying to grapple with these questions, it is useful first to review the history of vaccination, to understand how it has revolutionised modern medicine and the implications of vaccine hesitancy.

Smallpox, vaccination, and the rise of counter-vaccine movements

The history of vaccination is often traced back to the British scientist Edward Jenner, who in 1796 inoculated an eight-year-old boy, James Phipps, with cowpox pus from a lesion on the hand of Sarah Nelmes, who worked as a milkmaid. Jenner did this because it had been observed that milkmaids, women such as Nelmes who milked cows, seemed to rarely contract smallpox. Though few of us are concerned with smallpox today, it was one of the deadliest infectious diseases in human history. Described as the "Greatest Killer," smallpox was an incredibly painful sickness, resulting in the death of between 20–30% of all people who contracted it, and causing significant scarring and even blindness in survivors.[11] With this scourge in mind, Jenner postulated that milkmaids were shielded from smallpox because they had first been exposed to cowpox; a disease that resulted in similar but relatively benign symptoms. After taking fluid from cowpox pustules on a young milkmaid, Jenner inserted it into incisions that he had made on the boy's hands. The boy developed mild symptoms but then recovered, after which Jenner completed the same procedure using smallpox matter. Incredibly, no smallpox symptoms developed in the boy. Jenner's technique derived the name "vaccination" from the Latin word for cow, *vacca*.[12]

Although Edward Jenner is credited with ushering in our modern understanding of vaccination, the factual accuracy of his legendary medical story involving a milkmaid has since been questioned by historians.[13] It has also been recognised that Jenner was not the first person to use cowpox materials to combat smallpox. An English farmer named Benjamin Jesty, for instance, had already recorded performing a similar procedure 22 years before Jenner conducted his famous milkmaid experiment.[14] Additionally, many fundamentals of inoculation that underpinned Jenner's procedure had been previously recognised by others. For example, it had already been observed that many survivors of infectious diseases were immune to reinfection from the same ailments. *Variolation*, the practice of administering materials taken from smallpox blisters on infected individuals to non-infected patients to generate immunity, had also been established throughout different regions of the world. There were reports of such procedures being practised in Africa, China, India, and Turkey well before Jenner's 18th century test.[15]

Nevertheless, Jenner led the way in establishing vaccination's official scientific standing, and he also became the procedure's top populariser. As a result, it was knowledge of Jenner's cowpox trials that would eventually spread throughout the world, and the Harvard professor Benjamin Waterhouse later became the first to test it in the USA by employing the technique on his own children. In the 19th century, Louis Pasteur then revolutionized medicine by applying vaccination principles to produce lab-made vaccines to prevent bacterial and viral infections, including developing a vaccine for rabies. The 20th century then witnessed the creation of large-scale vaccine production techniques, and by the end of the 1900s researchers had developed individual vaccines for over 20 infectious diseases. These included vaccines for diphtheria, tetanus, anthrax, cholera, typhoid, tuberculosis, polio, measles, mumps, and rubella. Following on from such advancements, 183 years after Edward Jenner's vaccination experiment, the World Health Assembly, which is the decision-making body of the World Health Organization (WHO), officially declared that smallpox had finally been eradicated in 1979.[16] This milestone was described as the "world's most triumphant achievement in public health."[17]

Even so, the story of smallpox and vaccinations is not only a narrative about combating devastating, life-threatening illnesses. It is also a tale that involves a parallel rise of vocal opposition to vaccines, which erupted not long after widespread, government-initiated vaccination drives began in the early 1800s.[18] After Jenner demonstrated the usefulness of the cowpox-smallpox vaccination technique, the United Kingdom's government introduced the Vaccination Act of 1840. The Act delivered free vaccinations to the public, while it also made the comparatively riskier procedure of smallpox variolation illegal. Following on from this, the Vaccination Act of 1853 rendered vaccination mandatory for children up to three-months-old, wherein failure to comply resulted in a fine or even imprisonment. A series of additional Vaccination Acts were successively introduced in ensuing decades, which further consolidated and updated UK laws around compulsory vaccination and the types of penalties given to citizens for non-compliance.[19] Protests were launched in response to the 1853 Act, and the Anti-Vaccination League was founded in London. In 1867, the Anti-Compulsory Vaccination League was then established, and its members contended that mandatory vaccination policies violated people's personal freedoms.

Throughout the 1870s and 1880s numerous antivaccination publications were drafted and distributed across Great Britain, while new antivaccination organisations were also initiated across Europe.

On the other side of the Atlantic, in the USA, protesters against vaccination mandates were forming their own opposition groups. The Anti-Vaccination Society of America was formed in 1879, followed by the establishment of the New England Anti-Compulsory Vaccination League in 1882, as well as the Anti-Vaccination League of New York City in 1885. Such American organisations distributed antivaccination publications critical of compulsory vaccination policies, and they were successful in having mandatory vaccination laws repealed in several states throughout the country by challenging them in US courts. Along with complaints that obligatory vaccination policies infringed upon civil liberties and personal health choices, 19th century counter-vaccine claims in the US involved religious objections to the animal origins of vaccination materials, overt distrust in medicine, and scepticism about the effectiveness of the procedure itself.[20] Conspicuously, many of these very same grievances remain at the heart of modern antivaccination arguments, and they continue to be identified as sources of present-day vaccine hesitancy. What also unites historical and contemporary arguments against vaccination is that they have commonly been based on misunderstandings and misinformation about vaccines. This includes recurrent misconceptions about how vaccination works and the nature of vaccine ingredients, as well as miscalculations about the safety and necessity of vaccines. For this reason, it is essential to outline the basic science of vaccines, including their safety and effectiveness.

How do vaccines work?

In basic terms, vaccines harness your natural immune system by training your body how to recognise and then combat pathogens. Pathogens are disease-causing agents, including viruses, bacteria, fungi and parasites, that can lead to illness, injury, or death.[21] Every day, we come into contact with a legion of pathogens, and our immune systems are persistently defending our bodies against these invaders to stop us from becoming ill. The first line of defence against pathogens is described as the *innate immune system*. This includes chemical barriers that prevent infection, as well as our skin, the linings of our lungs and the digestive tract, which function as physical barriers to keep pathogens from invading the body. This innate immune system is also composed of certain white blood cells that guard the body from pathogenic assault.[22] Cumulatively, the innate immune system negates many potential pathogens, and it is nonspecific in nature, serving as a general defence barricade against entry into the body.

The most common variety of innate immune system white blood cells are *neutrophils*, which circulate in the bloodstream and only survive for a few days. When these cells identify a pathogen, they surround and ingest it. The innate immune system also includes *macrophages*, pathogen-engulfing white blood cells that live much longer than neutrophils. Macrophages are particularly important because they activate inflammation within the body, and they secrete signals to recruit other immune cells to the area. The innate immune system is also comprised of *natural killer cells*, which attach themselves to cells infected with viruses, as well as tumour cells, and then release chemicals to destroy the tissue. *Dendritic cells* of the innate immune system have threadlike tentacles to capture pathogens, which they then break apart and present to other immune cells to stimulate increased immune responses. These cells are vital because they activate another level of protection termed the *adaptive immune system*.

The adaptive system operates beyond the innate immune system's non-specific defences, for more precise, aimed action against specific pathogens. It works in concert with the innate immune system, and can detect unique molecular parts of pathogens, or molecules in the toxins that a pathogen can produce. These specific molecular parts of pathogens, or pathogenic toxins, are called *antigens*.[23] Every pathogen is composed of a unique set of building blocks, such as proteins and sugars, or nucleic acids like DNA. These individual building blocks, which can be recognised by the immune system to stimulate an immune response, are antigens. When the innate immune system's white blood cells, especially the dendritic cells, identify an antigen, they muster into action the adaptive immune system's own set of white blood cells.[24] The adaptive immune system's two primary types of cells include *T-cells* and *B-cells*. The T-cells essentially control and direct the adaptive immune system's more targeted responses, and they can also kill cells infected by pathogens. B-cells, which are activated by T-cells, are crucial because they manufacture *antibodies*. Antibodies are complex proteins, which serve as molecular weaponry that can lock onto specific antigens to neutralise them. Antibodies can also attach to pathogens and mark them for destruction by other white blood cells.

When the combined activities of the immune system fight off a pathogen, numerous activated white blood cells expire during, or shortly after the pathogenic invader has been destroyed. Yet, what is remarkably important about the adaptive immune system is that a small number of T-cells and B-cells remain in the body long-term. These are named *memory cells*, and they can recognise and target a specific antigen from a previous infection using receptors on their cell surfaces. Such cells can remain on guard for years, or even for the life of an individual, to provide long-lasting defence from reinfection.[25] Consequently, when someone is exposed to a pathogen that their memory cells are already primed to recognise, the memory cells will quickly trigger the immune system for an efficient, heightened, and more sustained defensive response. This can mean that some individuals may not express any symptoms when they are re-exposed to a pathogen that the immune system has previously fought off, or they could experience less severe symptoms over a shorter duration when compared to first-time exposure.

If a person has an immune system with memory cells that can recognise and mount a faster response to specific antigens, that individual sustains immunity to such antigens. The result is that the body can then destroy the related pathogen before it can cause disease, or, fight the infection to the degree of significantly reducing the span and severity of disease symptoms. Critically, this basic understanding of the immune system is fundamental to grasping how vaccines function, and why they are such a momentous medical intervention. This is because while our immune system is an extraordinarily complex and effective defence apparatus, which is constantly operating to keep us safe, some pathogens can overwhelm or evade our immune responses. Depending upon the pathogen, this can result in severe illness, injury or death before our bodies have the time to fight them off and develop memory cells. Vaccination for specific pathogens prevents that from happening. This is because vaccines safely introduce antigens into our bodies, though controlled exposure to a dead or weakened version of the pathogen, or only part of the pathogen, or even deactivated toxins that pathogens can produce. In its weakened state, a pathogen generally cannot replicate and spread throughout the body to cause the symptoms associated with natural exposure. Additionally, only parts of a pathogen, or deactivated pathogenic toxins, are also unlikely to result in adverse reactions. Even so, an introduced controlled antigen in a vaccine can still train the active immune system to fight off a natural infection.

The immune system learns to recognise the antigenic molecules in a vaccine as an invader, resulting in memory cells that are readied to know how to deal with them in the future. A vaccine accomplishes this without requiring that people be exposed to a full-scale infection from an active pathogen. In the end, what is fundamental is that natural infections and vaccines are both stimulating the *same* immune system defence responses. However, with a vaccine the body can acquire an adaptive memory cell outcome without having to endure or risk the potentially debilitating, and sometimes life-threatening, consequences of the disease itself.[26]

Types of vaccines

Though all vaccines train the immune system to fight pathogens by introducing antigens into the body, there are currently six major types of vaccines that have been developed that do this in somewhat different ways.[27] It is helpful to appreciate this diversity of vaccines, in order to understand the ways that each variety coaches our natural immune systems to fight off disease.[28] Basic knowledge about vaccine types is also vital because not everyone may be as aware of the range of vaccines on offer, while common misunderstandings and misinformation about vaccines often skew and overlook how different vaccines function. The assortment of commercially available vaccines includes the following.

Live attenuated vaccines

This class of vaccines contain a debilitated living version of the bacteria or virus that they are designed to produce immunity against. The pathogens are weakened in a laboratory so that they are unlikely to spread and result in symptoms. For instance, though naturally occurring viruses can reproduce thousands of times in the body during an infection, weakened viruses in live attenuated vaccines usually reproduce fewer than 20 instances. Since these types of vaccines introduce a live pathogen, they mimic natural infections and elicit relatively strong immune responses that often result in life-long immunity after only one or two doses. However, because they contain live pathogens, these kinds of vaccines are not given to people with immune deficiencies, including those with AIDs or patients undergoing cancer treatment. Live attenuated vaccines must also be kept refrigerated to prevent the weakened pathogens from dying. Examples of such vaccines include measles, mumps, and rubella vaccines, as well as vaccines for varicella, known as chickenpox.[29]

Killed/inactivated vaccines

These vaccines contain pathogens that have been killed by chemicals, heat, or radiation. The body can acquire immunity from the dead remains, as they still contain key antigens that allow the body to learn how to defend itself against a live infection. Unlike live attenuated vaccines, inactivated vaccines are easier to store and are safer for people with weakened immune systems because they contain no live pathogens. On the other hand, such vaccines frequently require several booster shots to fully instruct the immune system to defend the body against natural infection, since a dead pathogen is less effective at simulating a natural infection than are weakened living pathogens. Examples include Hepatitis A, rabies, and inactivated poliovirus vaccines.[30]

Subunit vaccines

These contain only an antigen component of a pathogen, rather than a whole weakened, or killed pathogen. The antigens can stimulate and train the immune system to combat a live pathogen. An ingredient called adjuvants are often required in these vaccines to help provoke the immune system, because antigens alone frequently do not elicit a sufficient reaction to result in long-term immunity. Adjuvants are vaccine ingredients that amplify the immune system's response to antigens. Since this variety of vaccine incorporates antigens rather than a live pathogen, the risk of side effects is low, and subunit vaccines can be given to people with immune deficiencies. However, identifying exactly which antigens can be used to develop immunity against a whole living invader often proves to be difficult, and subunit vaccines can only be made for certain pathogens. Vaccines for Hepatitis B, Haemophilus Influenzae Type B (Hib), Human Papillomavirus (HPV), and Meningococcal are all examples of subunit vaccines.[31]

Toxoid vaccines

Such vaccines utilise deactivated versions of toxins that are secreted by some bacterial pathogens. Such toxins are responsible for the symptoms of certain diseases, and they can be deactivated with formaldehyde (Chapter 4). The disease-causing bacteria are grown in a lab to cultivate the toxin, and once the toxin is deactivated, and now called a *toxoid*, it is filtered for use in a vaccine. The deactivated toxoid proteins are similar enough to the natural toxic variety that they induce immune responses that train the body to fight the disease's toxins in the future. Toxoid vaccines tend to be very stable and less sensitive to changes in temperature, humidity, or light, but as with subunit vaccines, they often require several doses, as well as adjuvants, to trigger the sufficient immune responses needed for long-lasting protection. Examples of this type of vaccine include vaccines for diphtheria and tetanus.[32]

mRNA vaccines

This variety of commercially available vaccines utilises fragments of a virus's genetic code called *messenger ribonucleic acid* (mRNA). In 2020, the first mRNA vaccine to be approved for use on humans was the Pfizer-BioN-Tech COVID-19 vaccine, which made headlines around the world in the midst of the coronavirus pandemic. Importantly, mRNA is a molecule that puts DNA instructions into action by telling cells what proteins to build. Put simply, the mRNA acts as a protein-coding template in cells. Proteins are the main component of bones, muscles, and other organs that make up our bodies, as well as being the building-blocks of viruses.[33] Viruses cannot make their own proteins, and they cannot replicate themselves independently from a host cell. Viruses inject their own DNA or RNA into host cells. The infected cells then synthesize the virus parts, which subsequently self-assemble into more viruses.[34] When the infected host cells break down, the viruses that they produced can spread to infect more cells. In the case of mRNA vaccines, a small section of a virus's mRNA is produced for the vaccine. This mRNA sequence codes for only one fragment of a virus's proteins. When the mRNA from the vaccine is introduced into human cells, the cells synthesize that protein, and then the immune system learns to combat it, providing future immunity from an actual virus.[35]

Notably, the mRNA does not combine with the DNA of a host cell, as it does not enter the cell's nucleus where the DNA is kept. It also degrades after the coded protein has been made. Since mRNA breaks down quickly, some mRNA vaccines need to be kept at low temperatures, which can make transport and storage difficult. To delay degradation, the mRNA strand is incorporated into other molecules or wrapped within fats.[36]

Viral vector vaccines

This variety of vaccine also made headlines during the COVID-19 pandemic, because the University of Oxford/AstraZeneca COVID-19 vaccine is based on this technology. A viral vector vaccine uses an altered version of a different virus than the pathogen against which the vaccine is immunising people. The modified virus functions as a vector, or a transport system, that delivers a piece of the genetic material from another virus into a vaccinated person's body.[37] While live attenuated and killed/inactivated vaccines use a weakened or an inactivated form of the target pathogen to elicit an immune response, viral vector vaccines use a completely different virus to deliver another virus's genetic material. The University of Oxford/AstraZeneca vaccine, for instance, uses a weakened and harmless chimpanzee adenovirus as the vaccine vector.[38] A gene which codes for the SARS-CoV-2 virus spike protein is added to the debilitated adenovirus vector, and this vector then delivers the COVID-19 gene to human cells. The viral vector uses this gene to synthesize the COVID-19 virus spike protein with the host cell's machinery, and the spike antigen is then displayed on the infected cell's surface.[39] The COVID-19 virus spike triggers an immune response, and trains the body to fight future infection from the actual COVID-19 virus. An advantage of viral vector COVID-19 vaccines is that they can be stored at normal refrigerator temperatures, which makes them easier to ship and administer. They are also relatively cheap to manufacture. However, people may have existing levels of immunity to the virus vector itself, which means that the immune system may attack the vector and reduce the vaccine's effectiveness.[40] This is why uncommon viruses, or viruses found in other species such as chimpanzees, are used in their development.

Vaccine ingredients

In addition to having a basic grasp of the types of vaccines utilised today, it is also valuable to gain a general understanding about what ingredients are employed in vaccines. This knowledge is essential when considering vaccine hesitancy, because throughout history vaccination uncertainties have frequently been linked to worries about such ingredients. Numerous counter-vaccine allegations and rumours, for example, revolve around the apparent dangers that vaccine ingredients are said to pose. For that reason, it is advantageous to obtain an elementary awareness of the main components of vaccines, and to understand why these ingredients are used to ensure their safety and medical effectiveness. These ingredients include the following.

Antigens

As noted above, antigens are the building blocks of pathogens, which are recognised by the immune system to trigger an immune response. They represent an active component of vaccines, which bring about immunity in vaccine recipients. Vaccines for different pathogens contain separate sets of antigens associated with the specific disease they are designed to produce immunity against. Antigen ingredients also vary according to the type of vaccine. Live attenuated vaccines and killed/inactivated vaccines contain a whole pathogen in either a weakened or a dead state. Subunit vaccines, toxoid, and mRNA vaccines on the other hand may include only specific antigen molecules, a deactivated toxin, or a piece of mRNA, rather than a complete pathogen.

Adjuvants

These are ingredients that function to intensify and help target the body's immune response against vaccine antigens. They do this by keeping the antigen close to the injection site, and by attracting immune cells to the area. Killed/inactivated vaccines and subunit vaccines require adjuvants to suitably alert the immune system of the antigen introduced to the body via the vaccine. The adjuvant does this by stimulating a stronger, and more extended immune response indicative of a reaction to a live pathogen. Since adjuvants boost immune responses, adjuvants usually result in lower quantities of an antigen being required per dose of a vaccine. In most cases, adjuvants are mineral salts such as aluminium hydroxide, aluminium phosphate, potassium aluminium sulphate, and calcium phosphate, which have well established safety track records (Chapter 4).[41] Other adjuvants include naturally occurring oil-in-water emulsions, as well as fats taken from the surface of bacteria.[42]

Expedients

This class of ingredient consists of vaccine ingredients other than the antigen and adjuvant active components, which are utilized during vaccine production, or which are present in the finished product to maintain the vaccine's quality and potency. Expedients include the following varieties of ingredients:

- *Buffers*. These are used to preserve the pH balance of vaccines. The most commonly used buffer is simply sodium chloride, otherwise known as salt.
- *Diluents*. These consist of liquids added to dilute vaccines to a proper concentration prior to their use. The diluent is usually sterile water or a sterile saline solution.

- *Preservatives.* These ingredients are added to vaccines to prevent fungal or bacterial contamination. The most widely used vaccine preservatives have included 2-phenoxyethanol, phenol, and thimerosal. 2-phenoxyethanol is metabolised in the human body and it is commonly found in baby care products as well as eye and eardrops. Phenol, an aromatic alcohol sometimes used in cosmetics, is seldom employed as a vaccine preservative, while thimerosal is a mercury-derived compound that was once used in healthcare products but is less common in vaccines today (Chapter 4).

- *Stabilizers.* These are additives that conserve vaccine effectiveness while in storage. They prevent chemical reactions from occurring and can stop vaccine components separating from each other. Stabilizers also keep vaccine elements from sticking to the sides of storage vials. Some examples include the sugars lactose and sucrose, as well as the amino acids, or amino acid salts glycine or monosodium glutamate. Proteins from baker's yeast or cow serum are sometimes also employed as stabilizers, as well as bovine and porcine gelatin.

- *Surfactants.* This type of ingredient lowers the surface tension of a vaccine's liquid to help keep particles from clumping together and settling at the bottom of vials. They are frequently derived from sorbitol, a sugar alcohol that is often used as a food sweetener.

- *Trace components.* These include small quantities of substances used in the production process of vaccines, and they are present in minute quantities measured in parts per million, or parts per billion of a total vaccine. Trace components vary depending upon the vaccine being manufactured. They can include antibiotics to ensure that bacterial contamination does not occur, as well as cell culture mediums and egg proteins used to grow antigens, formaldehyde when it is employed to deactivate toxins from bacterial pathogens, and yeast.

Why are vaccines important?

Within the gamut of historical and present-day misconceptions about vaccines, there frequently appear enduring questions about whether vaccines are truly necessary. A connected question has also been, why are vaccines still important? To address these queries, it is worthwhile to consider both the individual benefits of vaccination, as well as *herd immunity*. With regard to individual benefits, we can turn to the related ideas of *proactive medicine* and *preventative medicine*, which are often described in contrast with *reactive medicine*. The term proactive medicine has been highlighted in popular media, while also being a serious academic research topic. The aim of preventative medicine is the absence of disease; to avoid disease before it starts, or, halting a disease before it can result in complications after onset.[43] Rather than seeking to cure people reactively *after* they become ill, preventative medicine seeks to keep people from becoming unwell in the first place. Despite such noble goals, preventative medicine is not without its challenges. For instance, some preventative healthcare efforts could potentially be seen as being too expensive, where there might be better value in supporting reactive medicine for certain diseases. Furthermore, various proactive activities can be deemed too time costly for each patient in respect to the benefits of their preventative outcomes.

In taking all this into account, vaccines represent an exemplar case of successful preventative medicine, which is a central reason why they are still vital to public health. Plus, with respect to preventative health benefits, vaccines are most often thought of in terms of their swift impact in bestowing immediate protection for individuals from serious diseases. At the same time, together with the short-term benefits for individuals in preventing infection now, vaccines also avert long-term, lingering, and future complications that can arise from such viruses as Hepatitis B or C. Various pathogens like these can cause dormant and ongoing infections that result in not only immediate illnesses, but chronic damage to organs, including cirrhosis of the liver, as well as leading to other complications such as cancer.[44]

Yet the preventative health benefits of vaccines go beyond even the immediate and long-term protection that they supply to individuals. This is because vaccines can also deliver community health advantages that are conceptualised through the idea of herd immunity.[45] Herd immunity, also referred to as *herd protection*, is an indirect safeguard against some pathogens for individuals in a community who cannot be vaccinated. This includes newborns who have not yet received available vaccines, people who cannot be vaccinated due to medical reasons such as being organ transplant recipients or patients undergoing cancer treatment, as well as individuals with weakened immunity like the elderly. Herd immunity occurs when enough people in a population are made immune to a disease, resulting in secondary protection for those who are not. By way of illustration, assume that there is a situation in which 80% of a population has been sufficiently vaccinated against a viral pathogen, which means that they now are immune to that virus. This would mean that 4 out of every 5 people who might be exposed to the virus may not contract it, and will then not spread it onward. This helps to contain the circulation of the pathogen. A vaccinated person's immune system knows how to fight possible infection, and therefore, the virus is less likely to be passed on in a community from vaccinated individuals to anyone else. This results in fewer chances that the virus will be transmitted to a vulnerable person who is not able to get vaccinated, or those who may be immunocompromised. Vaccinated individuals, therefore, serve as a secondary preventative immune barrier for susceptible people.

Depending on the pathogen, and how infectious diseases might be, it is often estimated that approximately 70% to 95% immunity needs to be achieved across a total population to attain herd immunity. Such protection may be difficult to accomplish and is unobtainable for diseases that are not spread from person-to-person, including tetanus. However, through population wide vaccination efforts and the processes of herd immunity, it has been possible to control for such pathogens as diphtheria, polio, rubella, smallpox, as well as numerous other diseases.[46] These results have demonstrated that vaccines are not only important for protecting vaccinated individuals. Vaccines also prevent other susceptible people from contracting potentially dangerous and life-threatening diseases. Therefore, while members of the public may not feel particularly at risk from a disease themselves, vaccination is still emphatically beneficial for the larger population, as it may protect others who are vulnerable.

In addition to the short and long-term benefits for individuals, as well as community-wide disease prevention, there are further collateral factors to consider. This includes the idea that the importance of vaccines can be further measured in terms of their wider economic impacts. Vaccination has been found to be one of the most cost-effective preventative health tools because, in part, vaccines reduce health service costs by eliminating the medical system's need to treat patients who would have otherwise been infected with diseases that can now be vaccinated against.[47] Vaccines cost healthcare systems far less money overall, because people do not contract the pathogens that they have been vaccinated against. This reduces or eliminates related expenditures that would have been allocated to treating patients in terms of the work hours of health practitioners, as well as paying for medical facilities and post-infection treatments.[48] A 2016 study, for example, estimated that non–vaccination amongst adults resulted in a yearly financial burden of $7.1 billion in the USA alone, due to health care costs and income loss that could have been avoided through vaccines.[49]

Researchers have further identified wider economic benefits to vaccinating. Financial evaluations have calculated that vaccines increase economic productivity in societies because they reduce financial drains that would have been caused by people being unable to work due to either their own sickness, or while caring for ill family members.[50] COVID-19 vaccines also resulted in colossal positive economic impacts, as they accelerated societal wide financial recovery in the SARS-CoV-2 pandemic.[51] Aside from economics data, there are also quality of life measures enhanced by vaccines. This is because people's wellbeing may be dramatically improved through the prevention of diseases that lead to illness and permanent disabilities. At the same time, fewer sick days for children results in better educational outcomes.

These many benefits also matter because the diseases that vaccines help prevent have not simply disappeared, even if people are rarely exposed to their repercussions in their day-to-day lives. For instance, numerous countries around the world had at one time officially eliminated such diseases as measles. Nevertheless, when vaccination rates subsequently dropped, these same nations witnessed measles outbreaks. Furthermore, many preventable diseases, such as polio, have the capacity to inflict severe morbidities and death. Though these pathogens may be rare in many nations, they have stubbornly endured. Accordingly, it is necessary to continue to keep vaccination rates high to prevent disease resurgences.

Ultimately, vaccines are still important because they represent one of the most cost-effective, successful forms of preventative medicine available, which reduce healthcare expenditures by averting immediate infections, as well as the effects of chronic disease and long-term complications. They also protect the vulnerable through herd immunity and can improve economic productivity.[52] Perhaps most importantly, they continue to be needed because vaccine preventable diseases still exist to this day. Nonetheless, despite these lines of reasoning, for some people there remains an additional question that must also be taken seriously: Are vaccines themselves unsafe?

Are vaccines safe? Correlations and monitoring

Many people have not witnessed the deadly effects of vaccine preventable diseases for themselves. As a result, they may not recognise such pathogens as being immediate dangers. Instead, individuals might consider the perceived risks of getting vaccinated to be a much greater health hazard. In fact, often it can be more likely for people to have heard a story about apparent vaccine-caused injuries than it is to have personally experienced the negative effects of a vaccine preventable disease. This reality is part of the preventative medicine challenge linked to the success of vaccination. This challenge is also tied to the fact that vaccines are given to healthy people to avert disease, unlike medicines that are given in response to an existing illness. With all this in mind, the related question remains: *What are the risks of getting vaccinated?*

Vaccines, like all medical procedures, can have side effects.[53] From the start, this is important to acknowledge. Even so, the vast majority of vaccine side effects are minor, and last for relatively short periods of time. The most common of these include redness and swelling around an injection site that can arise within hours of being vaccinated. Less common reactions include fevers and tiredness, sometimes occurring within 24 to 48 hours of vaccine receipt, or even after longer periods of time depending on the vaccine, which may include a rash or other symptoms related to an immune response resulting from the vaccine ingredients.[54] While side effects are associated with vaccines, it is also the case that occasionally feeling unwell following vaccination may not be related to the vaccine itself. For example, it is not uncommon for people to experience fevers, runny noses, or coughs. When someone develops such symptoms in the days or even weeks following getting vaccinated, it may be assumed that the symptoms were triggered by a vaccine, even though the symptoms may only be correlated but not caused by vaccination. At times it can be difficult to know whether a particular sickness genuinely resulted from a vaccine itself, or from incidental symptoms that correlate over time, by chance, with getting vaccinated. This is the problem of correlation, or coincidence, versus causation.

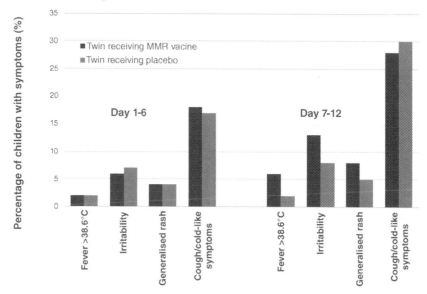

Figure 1.2 Comparison of common symptoms in a paired twin study, where one
twin received an MMR vaccine and the other received a placebo[55]

The puzzling nature of correlation versus causation and vaccines proved
to be such an important issue that it led a Finnish research team to conduct
a double-blind study with 581 sets of twins. One twin was given the
measles, mumps, rubella vaccine, known as MMR, and the other twin was
given a placebo.[56] Interestingly, the researchers found that between 1 to 6
days after being vaccinated, both twins experienced almost identical symptoms, even though only one of the siblings had received a vaccine with
antigens. Between 7 and 12 days, the MMR vaccinated twins did experience a statistical increase in various symptoms associated with the measles
live attenuated vaccine, such as fevers and rashes. Yet some of the twins
who only received a placebo also experienced similar symptoms, such as
fever, and, between both vaccinated and placebo-given twins there was no
statistical difference in cough and cold-like symptoms. Many of the most
customary symptoms associated with vaccines appeared in both groups of
twins, whether they received the true vaccine or the placebo. As a result,
the symptoms were a product of chance coincidences, in which the children
expressed correlative illnesses after being vaccinated. The vaccine, therefore,
could not have been the cause because one child did not actually receive it.
Despite this and other placebo-comparison studies, it is still common to hear
counter-vaccine claims, often made online, that no vaccine versus placebo,
or explicitly vaccine versus saline placebo safety analyses exist. However,
contrary to these assertions, numerous studies have employed placebos and
further concluded that adverse effects result primarily from correlational illnesses, and the result of chance. Such research has also involved the explicit

use of saline placebos versus vaccine tests, including saline placebos compared to adjuvants.[57]

Along with correlational analyses and research involving placebos, vaccine research has also been established on analyses that employ control groups, such as those comparing vaccinated populations vs unvaccinated or undervaccinated control groups.[58] Though counter-vaccine commentators frequently assert that such studies have never been conducted, there are a myriad of robust investigations involving these parameters. This includes long-term safety and side effects analyses, with samples ranging from thousands to millions of people, involving lengthy durations of monitoring over several years or even multiple decades.[59] There have also been extensive studies dedicated to researching the outcomes of giving vaccines together in combination.[60] Consequently, researchers from across the world have continued to test vaccines in combination, vaccines versus placebos, while conducting long-term studies on vaccine safety, as well as comparing groups of vaccinated and unvaccinated individuals.

Besides the preponderance of vaccine safety studies, the most central, reliable observations include copious amounts of data about the effects of vaccine preventable diseases, compared directly with the medical outcomes of society-wide vaccine uptake. This objective data involves comparing what is definitively known about the consequences of such diseases as diphtheria with vaccine side effects and immunisation outcomes. For example, longstanding medical observations found that of those who contract diphtheria, approximately 1 in 7 people die. By comparison, about 1 in 10 of DTaP/Tdap vaccine recipients will experience post-vaccination redness or swelling.[61] In the USA alone there were approximately 1,800 deaths per year from diphtheria from 1936 to 1945.[62] Reams of well-established data demonstrate that non-vaccination is the far riskier prospect. This is true, even when there may exist rare vaccine-related side effects.

Aside from more commonly observed, mild vaccine side effects, there have been more serious adverse effects reported. These include febrile seizures in children following receipt of the measles, mumps, and rubella vaccine. These are usually benign convulsions caused by a spike in body temperature.[63] What is important about such reactions, and their risks, is that the dangers of very serious complications from contracting measles are far greater than the hazards of side effects resulting from the MMR vaccine itself. To illustrate this point, it can be noted that out of 100,000 children who receive the MMR vaccine, approximately 25 to 34 may experience febrile seizures, which are not serious in nature.[64] That equates to 0.025 to 0.034% of children who are vaccinated. On the other hand, the risk of a child experiencing severe encephalitis caused by measles, with swelling of the brain that can also lead to seizures, occurs in approximately 1 in every 1,000 cases, or 0.1% of children. Chronic progressive brain inflammation, which is usually fatal, occurs in 1 in every 1 million cases of measles.[65] For these reasons, the proportion of side effects that might occur from the

MMR vaccine is far less significant than the measurable outcomes that occur if children contract the actual measles virus.

Such statistics are well established because research into vaccine safety, the monitoring of possible vaccine side effects, and analyses of vaccine efficacy are incredibly rigorous and ongoing. National regulatory authorities, such as the Food and Drug Administration in the USA, or the Therapeutic Goods Administration in Australia, and the European Medicines Agency in the EU, or the Medicines and Healthcare Products Regulatory Agency in the UK, evaluate and test vaccines prior to their use, and continue to monitor vaccines. Before vaccines can get to the point that they are distributed to the public, there are several safety hurdles that every developed vaccine must overcome.[66] First, there are preliminary laboratory analyses, which can involve testing a potential vaccine on mice. If a vaccine is proved safe in initial lab tests, it moves on to *Phase I* studies. These include initial trials using a small group of approximately 10–100 adults. Phase I testing seeks to identify any safety concerns in humans. If Phase I testing is passed, the vaccine moves on to a *Phase II* study. Phase II includes trials with larger groups of adult participants, usually involving several hundred people. In these studies researchers continue to look for any side effects. They also seek to identify whether the vaccine triggers the required level of immune response, while trying to pinpoint correct dosage amounts needed for the vaccine to be effective. If Phase II trials are acceptable, the vaccine moves on to *Phase III*. This involves testing the vaccine on 1,000–10,000 participants, to further identify if the vaccine is safe and effective in producing the required level of immunity to prevent the disease.

If each of these stages is passed, the vaccine then receives expert review by national regulatory agencies. Such agencies examine the cumulative research data to ensure that the vaccine's advantages far outweigh any possible disadvantages for the majority of people. If the vaccine passes this stage, it becomes approved for distribution. At this time, it then enters *Phase IV*, which involves continuing surveillance of the effects of the vaccine when given to the population. There are numerous national and international vaccine safety monitoring organisations that conduct such surveillance. For instance, in the USA the first level of monitoring is the Centers for Disease Control and Prevention, as well as the Food and Drug Administration, watch together watch for safety issues. American monitoring initiatives include the Vaccine Adverse Event Reporting System (VAERS), the Vaccine Safety Datalink established by the Centers for Disease Control and Prevention, and the Clinical Immunization Safety Assessment Project. Additionally, numerous other countries have their own vaccine monitoring agencies, such as the Therapeutic Goods Administration in Australia, the Canadian Adverse Events Following Immunization Surveillance System (CAEFISS), France's Agence nationale de sécurité du médicament et des produits de santé, Italy's Agenzia Italiana del Farmaco, and Japan's Ministry of Health, Labour and Welfare. Many other countries have additional layers of active monitoring on top of the ones listed here, which operate somewhat similarly to the Vaccine Safety Datalink in the US. For instance, in addition to Therapeutic Goods Administration in Australia, the country also features AusVaxSafety, which is a collaborative national vaccine safety system that actively monitors surveillance sites across the country. Likewise, Canada has the Immunization Monitoring Program ACTive, and the UK has the Clinical Practice Research Datalink.

Over and above national-level vaccine monitoring efforts, the World Health Organization's Global Vaccine Safety Initiative maintains partnerships with approximately 110 counties. This global monitoring network collates vaccine safety data from around the world. Additionally, The Institute of Medicine (IOM) has maintained 40 years of international vaccine safety reports and monitoring. The IOM is the Health and Medicine Division of the National Academies of Sciences, Engineering, and Medicine, and it is an independent, non-profit organisation that works outside of government to provide unbiased and authoritative advice to decision makers and the public.[67] In aggregate, each of the research stages and national and international regulatory bodies serve to ensure that vaccines are safe today and scrupulously monitored into the future. Moreover, the many studies analysing long-term vaccine safety, and the numerous safety monitoring organisations, involve different people, from a variety of backgrounds and cultures, working in countless independent labs across the globe. This reveals that vaccine safety maintains both international scrutiny and broad scientific consensus.

Additional safety questions

The testing and monitoring standards for vaccines are more rigorous than they are for most other types of medical intervention. In some cases, academic studies and surveillance standards have been set in response to rumours and enduring hesitations about vaccination safety. Unfortunately, explaining how stringent these international standards are is not necessarily enough to alleviate people's vaccine doubts. That is because vaccine hesitancy can be complicated and not always easy to address. It may have deep roots, wrapped around social connections, people's values, and their cultures, which can be tied to the subtleties of human behaviour and psychology. Such hesitancy may not be impacted by descriptions of vaccine safety standards and immunisation monitoring. With that actuality in mind, the next chapter will unpack the nuances of vaccine hesitancy in greater detail and reveal the primary reasons for less-than-optimal vaccine uptake.

Notes

1 WHO, "Ten Threats to Global Health in 2019," https://www.who.int/news-room/spotlight/ten-threats-to-global-health-in-2019.
2 Thomas Aechtner, *AVAXX101: Antivaccination and Vaccine Hesitancy* (edX, 2021).

3 Sachiko Ozawa, Ligia Paina, and Mary Qiu, "Exploring Pathways for Building Trust in Vaccination and Strengthening Health System Resilience," *BMC Health Services Research* 16, no. Suppl 7 (2016); Felix Gille, Sarah Smith, and Nicholas Mays, "Why Public Trust in Health Care Systems Matters and Deserves Greater Research Attention," *Journal of Health Services Research & Policy* 20, no. 1 (2015).
4 CDC, "Fast Facts on Global Immunization," Centres for Disease Control and Prevention, https://www.cdc.gov/globalhealth/immunization/data/fast-facts.html.
5 OED, "*Anti-Vaccinator, N.*" (Oxford University Press); Ngram, "Anti-Vaccination,Antivaccination," Google, https://books.google.com/ngrams/graph?content=anti-vaccination%2Cantivaccination&year_start=1800&year_end=2019&corpus=26&smoothing=3.
6 Timothy B. Gravelle et al., "Estimating the Size of 'Anti-Vax' and Vaccine Hesitant Populations in the US, UK, and Canada: Comparative Latent Class Modeling of Vaccine Attitudes," *Human Vaccines & Immunotherapeutics* 18, no. 1 (2022); Hannah Ritchie and Samantha Vanderslott, "How Many People Support Vaccination across the World?," https://ourworldindata.org/support-for-vaccination; Alexandre de Figueiredo et al., "Mapping Global Trends in Vaccine Confidence and Investigating Barriers to Vaccine Uptake: A Large-Scale Retrospective Temporal Modelling Study," *Lancet* 396, no. 10255 (2020); Wellcome, "How Much Does the World Trust Medical Experts and Vaccines?," Wellcome, https://wellcome.org/press-release/how-much-does-world-trust-medical-experts-and-vaccines; Justine Coleman, "Rates of Vaccine Skepticism Have Stalled," *Morning Consult*, https://morningconsult.com/global-vaccine-tracking/; Sarah Lane et al., "Vaccine Hesitancy around the Globe: Analysis of Three Years of WHO/Unicef Joint Reporting Form Data-2015–2017," *Vaccine* 36, no. 26 (2018); Jeffrey V. Lazarus et al., "A Survey of COVID-19 Vaccine Acceptance across 23 Countries in 2022," *Nature Medicine* (2023).
7 Eve Dubé, Maryline Vivion, and Noni E. MacDonald, "Vaccine Hesitancy, Vaccine Refusal and the Anti-Vaccine Movement: Influence, Impact and Implications," *Expert Review of Vaccines* 14, no. 1 (2015); Eve Dubé et al., "Mapping Vaccine Hesitancy—Country-Specific Characteristics of a Global Phenomenon," *Vaccine* 32, no. 49 (2014); Matthew Z. Dudley et al., "Words Matter: Vaccine Hesitancy, Vaccine Demand, Vaccine Confidence, Herd Immunity and Mandatory Vaccination," *Vaccine* 38, no. 4 (2020).
8 Heidi J. Larson et al., "Understanding Vaccine Hesitancy around Vaccines and Vaccination from a Global Perspective: A Systematic Review of Published Literature, 2007–2012," *Vaccine* 32, no. 19 (2014).
9 Adapted from: Noni E. MacDonald, "Vaccine Hesitancy: Definition, Scope and Determinants," *Vaccine* 33, no. 34 (2015): 4162.
10 Eve Dubé et al., "Vaccine Hesitancy: An Overview," *Human Vaccines & Immunotherapeutics* 9, no. 8 (2013); Dubé, Vivion, and MacDonald, "Vaccine Hesitancy, Vaccine Refusal."; Heidi J. Larson et al., "Measuring Vaccine Hesitancy: The Development of a Survey Tool," *Vaccine* 33, no. 34 (2015); Larson et al., "Understanding Vaccine Hesitancy around Vaccines and Vaccination from a Global Perspective: A Systematic Review of Published Literature, 2007–2012."; Barry R. Bloom, Edgar Marcuse, and Seth Mnookin, "Addressing Vaccine Hesitancy," *Science* 344, no. 6182 (2014); Dubé, Vivion, and MacDonald, "Vaccine Hesitancy, Vaccine Refusal."; Robert M. Jacobson, Jennifer L. St. Sauver, and Lila J. Finney Rutten, "Vaccine Hesitancy," *Mayo Clinic Proceedings* 90, no. 11 (2015); Catherine C. McClure, Jessica R. Cataldi, and Sean T. O'Leary, "Vaccine Hesitancy: Where We Are and Where We Are Going," *Clinical Therapeutics* 39, no. 8 (2017); Dudley et al., "Words Matter: Vaccine Hesitancy, Vaccine Demand, Vaccine Confidence, Herd Immunity and Mandatory Vaccination."; Daniel A. Salmon

et al., "Vaccine Hesitancy: Causes, Consequences, and a Call to Action," *American Journal of Preventive Medicine* 49, no. 6 Suppl 4 (2015); Melanie Marti et al., "Assessments of Global Drivers of Vaccine Hesitancy in 2014 - Looking Beyond Safety Concerns," *PLoS One* 12, no. 3 (2017); K. M. Edwards and J. M. Hackell, "Countering Vaccine Hesitancy," *Pediatrics* 138, no. 3 (2016).

11 Donald R. Hopkins, *The Greatest Killer: Smallpox in History* (Chicago: The University of Chicago Press, 2002).

12 Robert M. Wolfe and Lisa K. Sharp, "Anti-Vaccinationists Past and Present," *BMJ* 325, no. 7361 (2002).

13 Arthur W. Boylston, "The Myth of the Milkmaid," *New England Journal of Medicine* 378, no. 5 (2018).

14 R. Horton, "Myths in Medicine. Jenner Did Not Discover Vaccination," *BMJ* 310, no. 6971 (1995).

15 Ian Glynn and Jenifer Glynn, *The Life and Death of Smallpox* (London: Profile Books, 2005); Cary P. Gross and Kent A. Sepkowitz, "The Myth of the Medical Breakthrough: Smallpox, Vaccination, and Jenner Reconsidered," *International Journal of Infectious Diseases* 3, no. 1 (1998).

16 Scott Barrett, "The Smallpox Eradication Game," *Public Choice* 130, no. 1/2 (2007).

17 Frank Fenner et al., "Smallpox and Its Eradication," World Health Organization, https://www.ncbi.nlm.nih.gov/pmc/articles/PMC2491071/pdf/bullwho00076-0026.pdf.

18 Wolfe and Sharp, "Anti-Vaccinationists Past and Present."

19 Dorothy Porter and Roy Porter, "The Politics of Prevention: Anti-Vaccinationism and Public Health in Nineteenth-Century England," *Medical History* 32, no. 3 (1988).

20 Nadja Durbach, "'They Might as Well Brand Us': Working-Class Resistance to Compulsory Vaccination in Victorian England," *Social History of Medicine* 13, no. 1 (2000).

21 Kenneth Murphy and Casey Weaver, *Janeway's Immunobiology*, 9th ed., Immunobiology (New York, NY: Garland Science, 2017), 3.

22 Ibid., 3–11; Peter J. Delves et al., *Roitt's Essential Immunology*, 13th ed. (New York: John Wiley & Sons, 2017), 3–51.

23 Murphy and Weaver, *Janeway's Immunobiology*, 11–25; Delves et al., *Roitt's Essential Immunology*, 52–68.

24 *Roitt's Essential Immunology*, 16; Murphy and Weaver, *Janeway's Immunobiology*, 7.

25 *Janeway's Immunobiology*, 11–12.

26 Federica Sallusto et al., "From Vaccines to Memory and Back," *Immunity* 33, no. 4 (2010).

27 David Baxter, "Active and Passive Immunity, Vaccine Types, Excipients and Licensing," *Occupational Medicine* 57, no. 8 (2007).

28 Stanley A. Plotkin, Walter A. Orenstein, and Paul A. Offit, *Vaccines*, 6th ed., Stanley Plotkin, Walter Orenstein, Paul Offit, eds. (Edinburgh: Elsevier/Saunders, 2013).

29 R. E. Weibel et al., "Live Attenuated Mumps-Virus Vaccine. 3. Clinical and Serologic Aspects in a Field Evaluation," *New England Journal of Medicine* 276, no. 5 (1967); Raul Andino, Adam S. Lauring, and Jeremy O. Jones, "Rationalizing the Development of Live Attenuated Virus Vaccines," *Nature Biotechnology* 28, no. 6 (2010).

30 Iris Delrue et al., "Inactivated Virus Vaccines from Chemistry to Prophylaxis: Merits, Risks and Challenges," *Expert Review of Vaccines* 11, no. 6 (2012).

31 A. J. Zuckerman, "Subunit, Recombinant and Synthetic Hepatitis B Vaccines," *Scandinavian Journal of Gastroenterology* 20, no. S117 (1985).

32 Uwe Schauer et al., "Levels of Antibodies Specific to Tetanus Toxoid, Haemophilus Influenzae Type B, and Pneumococcal Capsular Polysaccharide in

Healthy Children and Adults," *Clinical and Vaccine Immunology* 10, no. 2 (2003); Janet A. Englund et al., "Maternal Immunization with Influenza or Tetanus Toxoid Vaccine for Passive Antibody Protection in Young Infants," *Journal of Infectious Diseases* 168, no. 3 (1993).

33 Patrick R. Murray, Ken S. Rosenthal, and Michael A. Pfaller, *Medical Microbiology*, 9th edition. (Philadelphia, PA: Elsevier, 2020), 362.

34 Ibid., 366–75.

35 Thomas Schlake et al., "Developing Mrna-Vaccine Technologies," *RNA Biology* 9, no. 11 (2012); Thomas Kramps and Jochen Probst, "Messenger RNA-Based Vaccines: Progress, Challenges, Applications," *WIREs RNA* 4, no. 6 (2013).

36 Norbert Pardi et al., "mRNA Vaccines — a New Era in Vaccinology," *Nat Rev Drug Discov* 17, no. 4 (2018); Thomas Kramps and Knut Elbers, *RNA Vaccines Methods and Protocols*, 1st ed. (New York: Springer, 2017).

37 Takehiro Ura, Kenji Okuda, and Masaru Shimada, "Developments in Viral Vector-Based Vaccines," *Vaccines* 2, no. 3 (2014).

38 "About the Oxford COVID-19 Vaccine," University of Oxford, https://www.research.ox.ac.uk/Article/2020-07-19-the-oxford-covid-19-vaccine.

39 "Understanding How COVID-19 Vaccines Work," Centers for Disease Control and Prevention, https://www.cdc.gov/coronavirus/2019-ncov/vaccines/different-vaccines/how-they-work.html.

40 WH Ng, X Liu, and S Mahalingam, "Development of Vaccines for SARS-CoV-2 [Version 1; Peer Review: 2 Approved]," *F1000Research* 9, no. 991 (2020).

41 Tom Jefferson, Melanie Rudin, and Carlo Di Pietrantonj, "Adverse Events after Immunisation with Aluminium-Containing Dtp Vaccines: Systematic Review of the Evidence," *Lancet* 4, no. 2 (2004).

42 Amy S. McKee and Philippa Marrack, "Old and New Adjuvants," *Current Opinion in Immunology* 47 (2017).

43 E. A. Clarke, "What Is Preventive Medicine?," *Canadian Family Physician* 20, no. 11 (1974).

44 G. Nebbia, D. Peppa, and M. K. Maini, "Hepatitis B Infection: Current Concepts and Future Challenges," *QJM* 105, no. 2 (2012); Stanislas Pol et al., "Hepatitis C: Epidemiology, Diagnosis, Natural History and Therapy," *Contributions to Nephrology* 176 (2012); Josep M. Llovet et al., "Hepatocellular Carcinoma," *Nature Reviews Disease Primers* 7, no. 1 (2021); Hashem B El-Serag, "Hepatocellular Carcinoma," *New England Journal of Medicine* 365, no. 12 (2011).

45 C. J. E. Metcalf et al., "Understanding Herd Immunity," *Trends in Immunology* 36, no. 12 (2015); Harunor Rashid, Gulam Khandaker, and Robert Booy, "Vaccination and Herd Immunity: What More Do We Know?," *Current Opinion in Infectious Diseases* 25, no. 3 (2012); Michael L. Mallory, Lisa C. Lindesmith, and Ralph S. Baric, "Vaccination-Induced Herd Immunity: Successes and Challenges," *Journal of Allergy and Clinical Immunology* 142, no. 1 (2018); T. H. Kim, J. Johnstone, and M. Loeb, "Vaccine Herd Effect," *Scandinavian Journal of Infectious Diseases* 43, no. 9 (2011); G. Gonçalves, "Herd Immunity: Recent Uses in Vaccine Assessment," *Expert Review of Vaccines* 7, no. 10 (2008); S. L. Pollard et al., "Estimating the Herd Immunity Effect of Rotavirus Vaccine," *Vaccine* 33, no. 32 (2015); Mohammad Ali et al., "Herd Immunity Conferred by Killed Oral Cholera Vaccines in Bangladesh: A Reanalysis," *Lancet* 366, no. 9479 (2005); Fine Paul, Eames Ken, and L. Heymann David, ""Herd Immunity"": : A Rough Guide," *Clinical Infectious Diseases* 52, no. 7 (2011); Daniel M. Musher, "Pneumococcal Vaccine — Direct and Indirect ("('Herd") ') Effects," *New England Journal of Medicine* 354, no. 14 (2006).

46 Mayo, "Herd Immunity and COVID-19 (Coronavirus): What You Need to Know," Mayo Clinic, https://www.mayoclinic.org/diseases-conditions/corona

virus/in-depth/herd-immunity-and-coronavirus/art-20486808; Katharine Hogg et al., "Immunity to Poliomyelitis in Victorians," *Australian and New Zealand Journal of Public Health* 26, no. 5 (2002); Tim Skern, ""100 Years Poliovirus: From Discovery to Eradication. A Meeting Report," *Archives of Virology* 155, no. 9 (2010); K. Lapinleimu and M. Stenvik, "Experiences with Polio Vaccination and Herd Immunity in Finland," *Developments in Biological Standardization* 47 (1981); Y. Ghendon and S. E. Robertson, "Interrupting the Transmission of Wild Polioviruses with Vaccines: Immunological Considerations," *Bulletin of the World Health Organization* 72, no. 6 (1994); Michael H. Le et al., "Prevalence of Hepatitis B Vaccination Coverage and Serologic Evidence of Immunity among US-Born Children and Adolescents from 1999 to 2016," *JAMA Network Open* 3, no. 11 (2020); Devin Razavi-Shearer et al., "Global Prevalence, Treatment, and Prevention of Hepatitis B Virus Infection in 2016: A Modelling Study," *Lancet* 3, no. 6 (2018); J. J. Ott et al., "Global Epidemiology of Hepatitis B Virus Infection: New Estimates of Age-Specific HBsAg Seroprevalence and Endemicity," *Vaccine* 30, no. 12 (2012); Kim, Johnstone, and Loeb, "Vaccine Herd Effect."; Pedro Plans-Rubió, "Evaluation of the Establishment of Herd Immunity in the Population by Means of Serological Surveys and Vaccination Coverage," *Human Vaccines & Immunotherapeutics* 8, no. 2 (2012); Alexandra Jablonka et al., "Tetanus and Diphtheria Immunity in Refugees in Europe in 2015," *Infection* 45, no. 2 (2017); Heather F. Gidding et al., "Immunity to Diphtheria and Tetanus in Australia: A National Serosurvey," *Medical Journal of Australia* 183, no. 6 (2005).

47 Caroline E. Wagner et al., "Economic and Behavioral Influencers of Vaccination and Antimicrobial Use," *Frontiers in Public Health* 8 (2020); Sam Ghebrehewet et al., "The Economic Cost of Measles: Healthcare, Public Health and Societal Costs of the 2012–13 Outbreak in Merseyside, UK," *Vaccine* 34, no. 15 (2016).

48 V. Remy et al., "The Economic Value of Vaccination: Why Prevention Is Wealth," *Value in Health* 17, no. 7 (2014).

49 Sachiko Ozawa et al., "Modeling the Economic Burden of Adult Vaccine-Preventable Diseases in the United States," *Health Affairs* 35, no. 11 (2016).

50 Bärnighausen Till et al., "Valuing Vaccination," *Proceedings of the National Academy of Sciences* 111, no. 34 (2014).

51 Nathan Fox et al., "The Value of Vaccines: A Tale of Two Parts," *Vaccines* 10, no. 12 (2022).

52 Katie Attwell, David T. Smith, and Paul R. Ward, "'If Your Child's Vaccinated, Why Do You Care About Mine?' Rhetoric, Responsibility, Power and Vaccine Rejection," *Journal of Sociology* 57, no. 2 (2021).

53 IOM, *Adverse Effects of Vaccines: Evidence and Causality*, ed. Clayton Ellen Wright, et al. (National Academies Press, 2012); Julia Stowe et al., "Investigation of the Temporal Association of Guillain-Barre Syndrome with Influenza Vaccine and Influenzalike Illness Using the United Kingdom General Practice Research Database," *American Journal of Epidemiology* 169, no. 3 (2009); David C. Wraith, Michel Goldman, and Paul-Henri Lambert, "Vaccination and Autoimmune Disease: What Is the Evidence?," *Lancet* 362, no. 9396 (2003).

54 W. Beyer et al., "Gender Differences in Local and Systemic Reactions to Inactivated Influenza Vaccine, Established by a Meta-Analysis of Fourteen Independent Studies," *European Journal of Clinical Microbiology and Infectious Diseases* 15, no. 1 (1996).

55 Adapted from: Heikki Peltola and Ollip Heinonen, "Frequency of True Adverse Reactions to Measles-Mumps-Rubella Vaccine: A Double-Blind Placebo-Controlled Trial in Twins," *Lancet* 327, no. 8487 (1986).

56 Ibid.

57   Suzanne M. Garland et al., "Safety and Immunogenicity of a 9-Valent HPV Vaccine in Females 12–26 Years of Age Who Previously Received the Quadrivalent HPV Vaccine," *Vaccine* 33, no. 48 (2015); Keith S. Reisinger et al., "Safety and Persistent Immunogenicity of a Quadrivalent Human Papillomavirus Types 6, 11, 16, 18 L1 Virus-Like Particle Vaccine in Preadolescents and Adolescents: A Randomized Controlled Trial," *Pediatric Infectious Disease Journal* 26, no. 3 (2007).

58   Roma Schmitz et al., "Vaccination Status and Health in Children and Adolescents Findings of the German Health Interview and Examination Survey for Children and Adolescents (Kiggs)," *Deutsches Ärzteblatt International* 108, no. 7 (2011); Natalie L. McCarthy et al., "Patterns of Childhood Immunization and All-Cause Mortality," *Vaccine* 35, no. 48 (2017); Phillip R. Pittman et al., "Long-Term Health Effects of Repeated Exposure to Multiple Vaccines," *Vaccine* 23, no. 4 (2004).

59   Allison L. Naleway et al., "Primary Ovarian Insufficiency and Adolescent Vaccination," *Pediatrics* 142, no. 3 (2018); Michael J. Smith and Charles R. Woods, "On-Time Vaccine Receipt in the First Year Does Not Adversely Affect Neuropsychological Outcomes," *Pediatrics* 125, no. 6 (2010); Jason M. Glanz et al., "Association between Estimated Cumulative Vaccine Antigen Exposure through the First 23 Months of Life and Non–-Vaccine-Targeted Infections from 24 through 47 Months of Age," *JAMA* 319, no. 9 (2018); Paulo S. Naud et al., "Sustained Efficacy, Immunogenicity, and Safety of the HPV-16/18 As04-Adjuvanted Vaccine: Final Analysis of a Long-Term Follow-up Study up to 9.4 Years Post-Vaccination," *Human Vaccines & Immunotherapeutics* 10, no. 8 (2014); Sara Miranda et al., "Human Papillomavirus Vaccination and Risk of Autoimmune Diseases: A Large Cohort Study of over 2 million Million Young Girls in France," *Vaccine* 35, no. 36 (2017); Roger P. Baxter et al., "Live Attenuated Influenza Vaccination before 3 Years of Age and Subsequent Development of Asthma: A 14-Year Follow-up Study," *Pediatric Infectious Disease Journal* 37, no. 5 (2018); Steven B. Black et al., "Lack of Association between Receipt of Conjugate Haemophilus Influenzae Type B Vaccine (Hboc) in Infancy and Risk of Type 1 (Juvenile Onset) Diabetes: Long Term Follow-up of the Hboc Efficacy Trial Cohort," *Pediatric Infectious Disease Journal* 21, no. 6 (2002); Shahed Iqbal et al., "Number of Antigens in Early Childhood Vaccines and Neuropsychological Outcomes at Age 7–10 Years," *Pharmacoepidemiology and Drug Safety* 22, no. 12 (2013); Linus B. M. D. M. P. H. Grabenhenrich et al., "Early-Life Determinants of Asthma from Birth to Age 20 Years: A german German Birth Cohort Study," *Journal of Allergy and Clinical Immunology* 133, no. 4 (2014); Outi Vaarala et al., "Rotavirus Vaccination and the Risk of Celiac Disease or Type 1 Diabetes in Finnish Children at Early Life," *Pediatric Infectious Disease Journal* 36, no. 7 (2017).

60   Zoe M. Rodriguez et al., "Concomitant Use of an Oral Live Pentavalent Human-Bovine Reassortant Rotavirus Vaccine with Licensed Parenteral Pediatric Vaccines in the United States," *Pediatric Infectious Disease Journal* 26, no. 3 (2007); S. Stojanov et al., "Administration of Hepatitis a Vaccine at 6 and 12 Months of Age Concomitantly with Hexavalent (DTaP–IPV–Prp~T–Hbs) Combination Vaccine," *Vaccine* 25, no. 43 (2007); Timo Prof Vesikari et al., "Immunogenicity and Safety of an Investigational Multicomponent, Recombinant, Meningococcal Serogroup B Vaccine (4cmenb) Administered Concomitantly with Routine Infant and Child Vaccinations: Results of Two Randomised Trials," *Lancet* 381, no. 9869 (2013); Timo Vesikari et al., "Safety and Immunogenicity of a Booster Dose of the 10-Valent Pneumococcal Nontypeable Haemophilus Influenzae Protein D Conjugate Vaccine Coadministered with Measles-Mumps-Rubella-Varicella Vaccine in Children Aged 12 to 16

Months," *Pediatric Infectious Disease Journal* 29, no. 6 (2010); Max Ciarlet et al., "Concomitant Use of the 3-Dose Oral Pentavalent Rotavirus Vaccine with a 3-Dose Primary Vaccination Course of a Diphtheria-Tetanus-Acellular Pertussis-Hepatitis B-Inactivated Polio-Haemophilus Influenzae Type B Vaccine: Immunogenicity and Reactogenicity," *Pediatric Infectious Disease Journal* 28, no. 3 (2009); Sylvia H. Yeh et al., "Immunogenicity and Safety of 13-Valent Pneumococcal Conjugate Vaccine in Infants and Toddlers," *Pediatrics* 126, no. 3 (2010); Heinz J. Schmitt et al., "Primary Vaccination of Infants with Diphtheria-Tetanus-Acellular Pertussis–Hepatitis B Virus– Inactivated Polio Virus and Haemophilus Influenzae Type B Vaccines Given as Either Separate or Mixed Injections," *Journal of Pediatrics* 137, no. 3 (2000).

61 "Comparisons of the Effects of Diseases and the Side Effects of Vaccines," Government of Western Australia Department of Health, https://ww2.health.wa.gov.au/Articles/A_E/Comparisons-of-the-effects-of-diseases-and-the-side-effects-of-vaccines.

62 Sandra W. Roush et al., "Historical Comparisons of Morbidity and Mortality for Vaccine-Preventable Diseases in the United States," *JAMA* 298, no. 18 (2007).

63 Sarah L. Sheridan et al., "Febrile Seizures in the Era of Rotavirus Vaccine," *Journal of the Pediatric Infectious Diseases Society* 5, no. 2 (2016); Lucy Deng et al., "Postvaccination Febrile Seizure Severity and Outcome," *Pediatrics* 143, no. 5 (2019); William E. Barlow et al., "The Risk of Seizures after Receipt of Whole-Cell Pertussis or Measles, Mumps, and Rubella Vaccine," *New England Journal of Medicine* 345, no. 9 (2001).

64 Christopher M. Verity, Rosemary Greenwood, and Jean Golding, "Long-Term Intellectual and Behavioral Outcomes of Children with Febrile Convulsions," *The New England Journal of Medicine* 338, no. 24 (1998); Jonas H. Ellenberg and Karin B. Nelson, "Febrile Seizures and Later Intellectual Performance," *Archives of Neurology (Chicago)* 35, no. 1 (1978); Barlow et al., "The Risk of Seizures after Receipt of Whole-Cell Pertussis or Measles, Mumps, and Rubella Vaccine."

65 Anne T. Berg, "Seizure Risk with Vaccination," *Epilepsy Currents* 2, no. 1 (2002): 16.

66 John Iskander et al., "Vaccine Safety," in *Vaccinology: Principles and Practice*, ed. W. John W. Morrow, et al. (Oxford: Blackwell, 2012).

67 IOM, *The Childhood Immunization Schedule and Safety: Stakeholder Concerns, Scientific Evidence, and Future Studies* (Washington, DC: The National Academies Press, 2013).

2 Why do people have vaccine hesitancy?

The previous chapter outlined how vaccines harness the natural mechanisms of the immune system. It also considered why vaccines are an incredibly safe, effective, and laboriously monitored means of preventing disease. Yet even though this is vital knowledge, it is also necessary to comprehend the reasons *why* some people can be apprehensive about immunisation. This is because if we truly want to address vaccine hesitancy, we need to first understand the social contexts and common concerns that are associated with vaccine refusal. It is also vital to grasp the sort of vaccine decision-making pathways that people tend to take, and the types of information that are often relied upon when questions about vaccines arise. For these reasons, studies have been conducted across the globe to identify external social and cultural contexts, as well as the inner rationale and motivations most frequently linked with people's vaccine choices. As it turns out, there are several reasons why different people, from different places and backgrounds, might not be getting vaccinated. People and communities are incredibly complicated, and so are the potential variables that can impact why vaccine uptake may be lower than optimal in various parts of the world.

The primary reasons for low vaccine uptake

There are seven overall factors that appear to be tied to lower likelihoods of getting vaccinated. These dynamics include an assortment of context-specific external social conditions, as well as underlying psychological tendencies. Importantly, these reasons are not necessarily mutually exclusive, and they often coincide with one another. The first of these seven factors is a key external concern that can be described as *access barriers*. Some people are not getting themselves and their family members vaccinated because, depending upon where they live in the world, it simply costs too much money. Alternatively, it may take too much time and effort to arrange vaccination appointments, with busy work schedules to manage. Life is hectic, and for some people the financial expenses and inconvenience of vaccinating can seem bothersome. What is important about access barriers is that low vaccine uptake is not necessarily a result of opposition to vaccines.

DOI: 10.4324/9781003312550-2

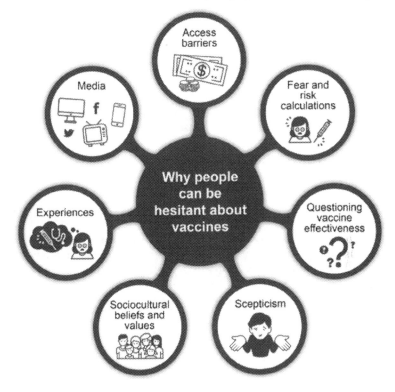

Figure 2.1 Seven reasons for low vaccine uptake

There can simply be too many obstacles in the way to make getting vaccinated an easy proposition.

A second general reason for less-than-optimal vaccination rates can be
described as *fear and risk calculations*. Some individuals are hesitant about
vaccines because they have heard about, and perhaps are afraid of, the
apparent dangers of getting vaccinated. Such risks include possible side
effects of vaccinations, stories about children developing autism because of a
vaccine, fears of vaccine ingredients, as well as a commonly held idea that
too many vaccines can overload a child's immune system (Chapter 4).
When such accounts of vaccine risks, and the thought of harm caused by a
vaccine, are weighed up against the idea that there may be a low danger in
getting infected by a vaccine-preventable disease, then some people calcu-
late that it is better not to be vaccinated at all. In tandem with risk calculations is the third reason for low vaccine uptakes described as *questioning
vaccine effectiveness*. At its core, this factor consists of scepticism about whether vaccines do in fact work (Chapter 3). Perhaps the true reason why we
do not see many vaccine-preventable diseases any longer is not so much due
to vaccines, a questioner may ask, but because of other societal changes

including better hygiene and clean water. Maybe the immunity we get from vaccines is not quite as robust as the immunity derived from fighting off a natural infection. Additionally, people may have heard that some vaccines, such as the annual flu shot, are not effective enough to be worth the bother.

Questioning vaccine effectiveness frequently overlaps with the fourth reason for low vaccine uptakes, described broadly as *scepticism*. This involves being sceptical about scientists, doctors and their medical advice, as well as distrusting healthcare authorities and governments enacting vaccination policies (Chapter 3).[1] Furthermore, people may also be particularly mistrustful of the pharmaceutical companies that produce vaccines, which can involve asking questions about BigPharma's financial motives, ethics, and the pharmaceutical industry's previous suspicious activity.[2] On the whole, many individuals are no longer prepared to simply follow a doctor's guidance or government policies without fact-checking for themselves first or talking to their friends and family. People can also question the vaccine experts and try to rely on their own perceived expertise and knowledge about their own wellbeing or their children's health. Research has found that this tendency can be associated with lower levels of intellectual humility.[3] Lower degrees of intellectual humility mean that people opposed to vaccines can be less likely to acknowledge that what they believe is wrong, while also being too overconfident in assuming that they know more than medical and scientific specialists. Altogether, the distrust associated with such perspectives can also overlap with conspiracy mindsets, and the sense that vaccines are part of a deliberate plot orchestrated by BigPharma, governments, doctors, and scientists to make money and even oppress the masses through vaccinations.[4]

A fifth reason for low vaccine uptakes is what can be broadly classified as *sociocultural beliefs and values*. An expansive spectrum of factors connected to personal philosophies and ideals, community values, and resistance to vaccination can be included within this wide-ranging variable. For example, people may value civic freedoms and personal autonomy in health decision-making. Consequently, mandatory vaccination policies may be viewed as an infringement upon citizen rights and self-determination. In a connected way, resistance to compulsory vaccination can also be associated with certain philosophical values and political ideologies, which may together espouse public liberties over mandatory government health policies. Resistance to vaccination may also be kindled because vaccines are interpreted to be unnatural, violating some people's desire to live a natural lifestyle and avoid unfamiliar chemicals. For others, certain religious doctrines and religious community connections can mutually impact the acceptance or refusal of vaccines. Importantly, one of the unifying features of all these different beliefs and cultural values is that they tend to be connected by social networks. Our values and beliefs do not occur in a vacuum, but they are given life in communities, as people are inclined to interact with others who share those same views. Such communities include people's family members, friends, as well as local or online groups who often maintain similar socio-cultural beliefs, values, and political viewpoints.

A sixth reason for low vaccine uptake includes *negative experiences*. When people have an unpleasant memory of getting vaccinated, or, if they have had poor interactions with healthcare practitioners when asking vaccine questions, they are more likely to reject future vaccinations. This might include an upsetting childhood experience of the pain and trepidation associated with getting immunised. It may also involve feeling snubbed by a healthcare professional who was perceived to be mocking a hesitant individual's vaccine fears about safety. People's first-hand experiences deeply shape how they view the world, and if individuals feel as though their questions and fears have been abruptly brushed off by a doctor, or if they feel as though they have been ridiculed by a professional for their hesitancy, it can cement negative vaccine attitudes.

Finally, the seventh potential factor that may affect vaccine uptakes includes *media influences*. Vaccination anxieties can be fuelled by disin-formation spread via media produced by vocal ardent vaccine deniers. This media is often online, shared across social media networks, and it can tap into many of the other factors outlined above that lead to low vaccine uptakes. For instance, such messaging frequently validates people's vaccine fears and perceptions of risk by telling stories of apparent vaccine injuries (Chapter 4). These messages recount a parent's experiences with what they presume is vaccine-caused damage in their children. Such media also fre-quently communicates to audiences that vaccines are ineffective, that man-datory vaccination policies infringe upon our personal freedoms, and they might emphasise that people should distrust vaccination authorities who are apparently conspiring to peddle vaccines for profit (Chapter 3). Notably, these messages can be surprisingly persuasive and psychologically sticky, which helps them spread vaccination myths and misinformation.

A central lesson that can be gleaned from these seven points is that the reasons why people can be hesitant about vaccines, and why some indivi-duals do not get vaccinated, can be complex. There may be multiple factors working in parallel to lessen vaccine uptake, which range from fear, values, past experiences, distrust, and media, as well as access barriers. Significantly, when it comes to barriers, for many people a lack of health cover, or the inability to take time off work, as well as problems with scheduling medical appointments or other access issues, might be preventing individuals from getting vaccinating.[5] Consequently, from the outset, policymakers and health providers should continually be seeking ways to reduce possible bar-riers wherever possible, because removing such obstacles could be an immediate way of boosting vaccination uptake (Chapter 5). Nevertheless, for other people, vaccine decision-making can be tied to several worries about safety, scepticism, social connections, and media influences, which can collectively result in a tangle of vaccine hesitations. This chapter will continue to unpack the myriad of social and psychological factors that may contribute to low immunisation uptake and vaccine hesitancy in more detail. In advance of that, however, it is important to consider exactly where people tend to turn for information when they have questions about vaccines.

Where do people turn for vaccine information?

When faced with vaccine concerns, many people's first source for answers and advice tends to be a local healthcare professional. Medical providers remain people's most trusted sources of vaccine information; this can include family doctors, nearby pharmacists, a child health or immunisation nurse, and paediatricians. However, many individuals also endeavour to seek out for themselves what they believe to be the "real truth" about vaccines.[6] Some parents, for instance, will simply not accept vaccination advice from healthcare providers without question.[7] Instead, they turn to the Internet for information, as well as relying upon the opinions of friends, relatives and close social networks.[8]

Such quests for truth can be provoked by the opinion that *real* data on vaccine safety and effectiveness is being supressed, or not freely given to the public by healthcare providers and pharmaceutical companies.[9] In this mindset, it is thought that conscientious citizens are forced to seek out the full details for themselves, including scouting online information.[10] In fact, studies indicate that a majority of people search for health information online, and that for some people, their primary source of vaccine information is the Internet.[11] This frequently involves using Google to find websites, social media posts, blogs, and online parenting forums that discuss vaccines.[12] Resistance to vaccination also seems to be more strongly associated with relying on the Internet, social media, and friends as sources for vaccine information, rather than authoritative, traditional suppliers of medical advice such as doctors and health officials.[13] Exposure to online vaccine misinformation has been correlated with greater immunisation hesitancy, and people who use the Internet to search about vaccines are more likely to perceive them as being unsafe.[14]

The link between vaccine rejection and a reliance on the Internet may seem unsurprising when considering the sheer quantity of online misinformation, and the ability of social media to amplify counter-vaccine myths.[15] Antivaccination websites and social media posts are often more numerous than are pro-vaccine messages, and they can appear in search engine results despite algorithms designed to limit the spread of misinformation.[16] Vaccine deniers can outperform pro-vaccinationists in terms of generating counter-vaccine websites and media posts, as well as by triggering greater user engagement and content sharing.[17] A 2020 analysis of Twitter posts, for example, found that antivaccination posts were reshared 7.4 times more than were pro-vaccine tweets.[18] These widespread antivaccine messages are also created by a relatively small number of so-called "superspreaders" who manipulate social media to circulate disinformation online.[19] One report concluded that up to 73% of all anti-vaccination content on Facebook, for example, originates from only twelve antivaccine campaigners.[20] Due to such activities, large numbers of information-seekers can encounter counter-vaccination sites and anti-immunisation social media posts simply because of the pervasiveness of such vaccine-rejecting materials.[21] Also, online antivaccination communications tend to be far easier to read, and they frequently contain more persuasive messaging than can be found in pro-vaccine websites.[22] Researchers have further documented the ways that persuasive anti-vaccination internet messages can have enduring effects on audiences, which capitalise on people's information obtaining proclivities. In fact, academics have warned that even very brief exposures to online counter-vaccination claims can have long-lasting negative influences upon immunisation attitudes and behaviours.[23]

People, therefore, often search for vaccination info online, where anti-vaccination messaging can be more prevalent than pro-vaccine internet sources. These widespread online antivaccination messages tend to be easier to read than pro-vaccine information, while counter-vaccine media are also filled with persuasive elements that can have enduring influences on the public. They are catchy, or cognitively "sticky", and are shared within networks of like-minded communities. What is also significant about the tendency to seek out info online, is that it can lead people to end up in vaccine-doubting *echo chambers*.[24] An echo chamber results from online selectivity effects, which involve individuals primarily searching out information and opinions that agree with their existing biases and beliefs, which can result in only connecting with likeminded people who have similar views to their own.[25] Social media and internet feeds are also algorithmically customised for users, to show them more items similar in relevance to those that they have already shown an affinity for.[26] Searching for and viewing counter-vaccine posts and videos can then lead to a tailored feed of similar content. Consequently, people may only encounter messages and claims that affirm and further amplify their pre-existing ideas and vaccine hesitancy.[27] Individuals then become cocooned within online networks that reject alternative views or data, which are populated chiefly by people echoing the same ideas, values, and sociocultural beliefs. Some people, therefore, only become exposed to online information that confirms their prior vaccine doubts, as well as other sociocultural values and perspectives that they already agreed with in the first place. If people were sceptical of vaccine safety before they began their internet searches, they may gravitate toward information, social media links, and sources with similar points of view. This can insulate them within networks that only reconfirm and express similar vaccine scepticism. Ultimately, this further entrenches vaccine doubts.

Echo chambers can occur offline as well. Beyond the Internet, individuals also tend to be socially attracted to, and to associate with, people displaying similar characteristics or cultural attitudes to those that they already hold.[28] We are inclined to interact with others who have the same political and cultural values, and we tend to accept the opinion of people with similar worldviews. If everyone in our local social network has vaccine doubts, then it is more likely that we too will have uncertainties, because we will primarily be exposed to the same viewpoints and information sources. We are disposed to agree with our close friends, family, and people in our social communities who we already see eye to eye with on other matters. In a nutshell, we have a propensity to accept ideas and data that confirm our existing biases, and we are more inclined to accept the opinions of people who have similar values and beliefs to our own. We can end up being insulated to contrary views and information, both when we are on the Internet seeking medical information, or offline in our close social networks discussing vaccines.

The information deficit myth

What is particularly notable about echo chambers is that misinformation that reinforces particular views can be circulated and recirculated within their closed confines. With that in mind, both vaccine hesitancy and anti-vaccination media usually have at their core fundamental misconceptions and vaccine misinformation. At the same time, it is also important to acknowledge that people frequently do not understand the complexities of vaccine hesitancy, while there are also several common miscalculations about how to best respond to vaccine doubts. This is because a common opinion, shared by many academics and medical practitioners, is that vaccination fears and mistaken beliefs about vaccines should be addressed by communicating more facts to the public. The assumption is that the problem of vaccine hesitancy is caused by a lack of information, which can be remedied by communicating additional data to people. This idea has been referred to as the *Information Deficit Model* of science communication. While it might seem logical, research has found that communicating scientific data does not necessarily work.

At the heart of the Information Deficit Model is the assumption that people are sceptical of scientific premises because they lack knowledge and have poor scientific literacy.[29] The deficit model has traditionally suggested that the solution then to erroneous beliefs about science, such as vaccines, can be found in supplying the public with more information, and making difficult to understand science more understandable. It has been understood that this will result in the acceptance of scientific ideas.[30] However, even though it might sound reasonable, the Information Deficit Model of science communication has run into problems. This is because studies have found that increasing people's factual knowledge and testable understanding of vaccines, for instance, does not necessarily translate into confidence in vaccination, or in improved immunisation behaviours.[31]

Surprisingly, trying to correct vaccine misinformation with scientific data can actually be counterproductive, leading to lower intentions to vaccinate.[32] This can be a difficult conclusion for people to accept, but strikingly, research has repeatedly found that an individual's understanding of the data and theory underlying consensus science, like vaccination, is often not a reliable indicator of the acceptance of those same scientific ideas.[33] In fact, studies have found that individuals opposed to vaccination demonstrate just as much, if not more knowledge about vaccines, as compared to the average person who supports them.[34] Knowledge is frequently not what makes the difference. As a result, when it comes to vaccine hesitancy, trying to change minds through the amplification of fact claims alone to correct misinformation is unlikely to be productive.[35]

An academic study succinctly concluded that there is "robust literature across disciplines to suggest that simply providing information often does not lead to people changing their views and may even create a dynamic in which a patient or a parent is actually less receptive to information a provider may impart."[36] Another group of researchers have likewise stated, "One striking aspect of the public's views of science is that general level of education, scientific knowledge, and science literacy are only modestly predictive of the public's general attitudes toward and trust in science."[37] This is because people are liable to make decisions about vaccines and other science not only on the basis of data and fact claims. Instead, people make such decisions against the backdrop of sociocultural influences, which are linked with their identity associations and personal values. Facts and science comprehension levels are clearly not the only ingredients that matter when it comes to the decision-making dynamics around vaccines. As Susanna Priest has rightly put it, knowledge "does matter," but it "is just not the only thing that matters, and often it is not the main issue when science and society appear to be in conflict."[38]

Certainly, researchers are not suggesting that trying to provide sceptical audiences with credible vaccine information is unimportant.[39] It will always be vital to get solid, intelligible, scientific vaccine data out to seeking publics, through online and offline channels. This is especially valuable because antivaccination misinformation is so prolific, which engenders the need for trustworthy, scientifically grounded data. Furthermore, many questioning parents do report that they would like more access to dependable vaccine information. It has to be recognised, however, that vaccination beliefs and behaviours are often driven by a number of psychological factors, along with people's social networks and connections, their political views, and other cultural considerations, that work in combination with an individual's scientific understanding of data. For example, social networks and social norms can greatly impact vaccine choices, because people tend to tailor their own behaviours to match up with the actions of their peers and members of the groups that they self-identify with (Chapter 5).

Individuals are also inclined to interpret and accept vaccination facts through the lens of cultural values rather than only via scientific facts.[40] It turns out that people tend to accept or reject vaccines, or any other science for that matter, based on the core values and beliefs held by the groups with which they personally identify. If people's family, friends, and local or online communities all insist that mandatory vaccination policies violate personal freedoms, or that vaccines are dangerous, they we will be more likely to question vaccination. Publicising scientific data is always important, but facts are accepted, rejected, and sometimes totally reinterpreted according to people's own social connections, beliefs and values. Accordingly, it must be acknowledged that an increase in data communication will not always bring success.

A pressing question then is: what should vaccine advocates and policymakers do if the Information Deficit Model is a myth? To start, it is crucial to accept that while being a venerable pursuit, simply increasing vaccine fact communications is not a silver bullet for countering vaccination hesitancy. It is also necessary to consider additional ways of reaching vaccine hesitant individuals, while bearing in mind the psychological dynamics that underpin vaccination decision-making. For that reason, this chapter will now consider common psychological factors that tend to influence the acceptance or rejection of vaccines.

Vaccination decision-making

Recall that there are seven general reasons for low vaccine uptakes which include the following elements:

1   Access barriers
2   Fear and risk calculations
3   Questioning vaccine effectiveness
4   Scepticism
5   Sociocultural beliefs and values
6   Experiences
7   Media

In considering these seven factors, it is important to emphasise that vaccination decision-making can differ greatly from person-to-person and community-to-community. Such decisions can vary according to cultural and social contexts, as well as people's varied experiences and backgrounds. Nevertheless, research has found that several common psychological factors tend to influence the vaccine acceptance. These psychological dynamics often overlap with each other, and they intersect directly with the seven general reasons for low vaccine uptakes.

1 Access barriers

Access barriers must always be taken into account when considering vaccine uptakes. However, the psychology around access barriers is not necessarily associated with vaccine hesitancy or zealous opposition to vaccination. Instead, such barriers encumber people's ability to get vaccinated, and they include decision-making dynamics around financial constraints, time commitments, work schedules, and vaccinations; where vaccine requirements can be side-lined by the demands of life and poor access being delivered by governments or healthcare systems. First and foremost, therefore, health providers and government policymakers should always be considering how to reduce access barriers for the public. Societal factors reducing vaccine uptake due to deficient access, and social interventions designed to mitigate such barriers, can frequently be more important than trying to bust anti-vaccination myths. This might include providing onsite vaccination drives at people's places of work, as well as actively reducing logistical and economic barriers inhibiting people from getting vaccinated (Chapter 5).

2 Fear and risk calculations

A Pain and disgust

When considering fear, it is important to bear in mind that anxiety about vaccination may involve more than just concerns about adverse side effects. This is because an initial psychological barrier to vaccinations includes people's fear of needles, and the immediate distress caused by that vaccination pain.[41] One study found that up to 63% of children and 24% of parents reported having such fears.[42] These injection phobias can be a strong enough to impede people from getting vaccinated.[43] Research has identified that the leading concern parents expressed about vaccines was the pain that their children would experience from getting vaccinated.[44] Though it might seem easy to dismiss such fears, people's apprehensions about vaccine-related pain can be an important decision-making driver. At the same time, people's underlying disgust with needles, hospitals, and blood, can also cause remarkably strong aversions to vaccination.[45] Consequently, added to fears about pain, some people are psychologically repelled by the thought of getting an injection into their bodies, and will avoid vaccines as a result.[46]

B Health intuitions

Health intuitions are commonly held impressions about the human immune system and health matters that can influence vaccine risk calculations. They include the belief that immunity gained from natural infection, rather than through a vaccine, results in stronger protection (Chapter 3).[47] These notions can also involve the idea that vaccines may overload a person's immune system.

It is not uncommon, for instance, for people to believe that this overloading may cause long-term harm to a child's body by damaging or disrupting the immune system's development, rather than boosting its ability to fight pathogens (Chapter 4).[48] Parents with children who have such conditions as allergies, asthma, eczema, and learning disorders have been found to express such worries.[49] These sorts of intuitions also include the impression that vaccines are an unnatural, artificial health option. Instead, good hygiene, nutrition, and a natural lifestyle are considered by some people to be better preventative health alternatives (Chapter 3).

C Risk perceptions

People are notorious for miscalculating risk. In vaccine decision-making this can involve attempts to gauge the likelihood of harm occurring if vaccines are avoided and comparing such possibilities with the perceived risks of getting vaccinated.[50] Decision-making may then be influenced in accordance with whether the perceived risks of contracting a vaccine preventable disease are assessed to be greater than the supposed hazards of getting vaccinated. As might be expected, parents tend to be more accepting of vaccines when the infectious diseases that vaccinations prevent are thought to have dangerous consequences.[51]

What complicates these calculations is that many individuals have not witnessed the detrimental effects of vaccine preventable illnesses for themselves. Risk perception can be further confused since vaccines are a pre-emptive health measure that stops infectious maladies from the outset. Consequently, it may be difficult for people to evaluate the true benefits of vaccination because, unlike most medicines used to treat sicknesses after they manifest, vaccines are designed to prevent an illness from occurring at all. Vaccines might then be thought of as something done to healthy people, rather a safe measure designed to keep healthy people safe, since their preventative effectiveness cannot be measured by the average person. It may also be the case that infectious diseases being vaccinated against, such as measles, are thought to be rather trivial maladies.[52] The rumoured stories of vaccine risks, on the other hand, can seem much more striking by comparison.

Finally, many parents tend to evaluate vaccine risks in relation to perceptions of their own children's health, over-and-above matters of population-wide safety.[53] Accordingly, if a parent believes that their child's health may be negatively impacted by a vaccine, that conviction can override concerns about public duty and the collective benefits of herd immunity.[54] In this way, vaccines can be assessed by some parents to be suitable for most people, but not for their own child because of existing health issues.

3 Questioning vaccine effectiveness

Doubts about the effectiveness of vaccines can be related to fear and risk calculations. People who question vaccine safety, and who believe that a vaccine preventable disease poses little risk, may further eschew immunising if they also suppose that a vaccine is not particularly effective in the first place.[55] Notably, questioning the effectiveness of vaccines is a common theme in antivaccination media, which involves disputing whether vaccines truly result in immunity (Chapter 3).[56] Such claims can insist that scientific evidence has demonstrated that vaccines played absolutely no role in the decline of infectious diseases.[57] These sorts of allegations have remained a persistent feature of counter-vaccine messages throughout history, and they are frequently stated in relation to health intuitions.[58] The health intuitions accompanying questions about vaccine effectiveness, discussed above, can assert that natural infections confer a more robust form of immunity than vaccines, as well as that other health measures, such as hygiene, have truly been responsible for disease declines.[59]

4 Scepticism

A Trust and distrust

One of the key factors in vaccine decision-making is whether people trust or distrust health providers, governments, and pharmaceutical companies.[60] Research has often reported that parents' decisions around vaccinating their children are impacted by levels of trust in the medical establishment, and vaccine choices vary depending upon who exactly people place confidence in for vaccine information.[61] Many parents respect their local healthcare practitioners and esteem the vaccine information that they provide. Others, however, are more inclined to trust friends and family, or anecdotal stories about vaccines from other parents or online voices over the advice of medical experts.[62] This is because some parents distrust official sources of vaccine information, while they tend to believe that fellow mothers and fathers are less biased.[63] "While there are many hurdles to vaccinating," concludes one study that analysed vaccine acceptance around the world today, "lack of trust in vaccines is an important barrier in some populations."[64]

B Conspiratorial beliefs

Conspiracy theories have been described as efforts "to explain some event or practice by reference to the machinations of powerful people, who attempt to conceal their role."[65] Importantly, at the core of many anti-vaccination messages are conspiratorial claims that vaccine-deniers are being censored by a powerful BigPharma-supporting cadre, which is hiding the unsuccessful and dangerous nature of vaccines for their own financial gain.[66] These conspiracy messages are infused with distrust narratives, and they can impact people's decisions.[67] Numerous studies have identified correlations between people's willingness to accept conspiracy theories and lower intentions to vaccinate, along with increased likelihoods of exhibiting anti-vaccine attitudes.[68] As the authors of one report concluded, antivaccine beliefs "are best thought of as part of a psychological propensity to believe in conspiracies."[69]

C Psychological reactance

In relation to feelings of distrust, some people also respond negatively to the idea that they are being coerced by a government through mandatory vac-cination policies. The sense that our vaccination choices are being forcibly limited can spark what has been described as *psychological reactance*. Psycho-logical reactance refers to a "set of motivational consequences that can be expected to occur whenever freedoms are threatened or lost."[70] According to the theory of psychological reactance, when a person feels as though their freedom of behaviour has been removed or restricted in some fashion, the "threat to or loss of freedom motivates the individual to restore that freedom."[71] It has been suggested that such reactance may be a key factor contributing to vaccine rejection.[72] In effect, people can resent being told what to think or how to act, especially by a government that they distrust, so they reject authoritative commands around vaccines.[73] This consideration is of particular relevance in countries like Australia, where families may be financially penalised if their children are not up to date in their immunisations.[74]

5 Community connections and cultural beliefs

A Social identity

An important predictor of many people's vaccination decisions is whether others closest to them, including those individuals they respect and identify with, are supportive of vaccination.[75] It is vital to recognise that most vac-cination decisions are made in the context of relationships with others.[76] People tend to shape their own behaviours and cultural beliefs to match up with the social norms of their peers, and the members of groups with whom they self-identify.[77] Additionally, antivaccinationists identify with each other as a social group, and such social identification can feel like a positive, psy-chologically advantageous group connection. This is because, along with "holding negative views toward vaccine safety, anti-vaxxers who socially identify with the group likely receive psychological benefits from belonging to a community, including increased self-esteem and a sense of community, by fulfilling their need to belong."[78]

Generally, if an individual's social identity, peer groups, and familial social norms are connected to questioning or rejecting vaccines, a person will also be inclined to have matching vaccine hesitancy. This can occur because a person may fundamentally agree with the opinions held by those around them, or, because it is socially advantageous to do so for the sake of one's reputation and community connections.[79] We are all social beings influenced by such group dynamics, one way or another, and social identity can be a powerful influence whether people are aware of it or not. At the same time, individuals tend to be socially attracted to, and to also associate with others who have similar cultural attitudes and views on health matters.[80] This tendency is called *homophily*, and it leads to people with vaccine hesitancy to socially cluster together in networks and make similar vaccination decisions together.

B Religious beliefs

For some individuals, religious communities represent significant social group influences. Religion has been identified as a potential global cause of vaccine hesitancy and immunisation refusal.[81] People most opposed to vaccines can, in some nations, be more likely to self-identify as being religious.[82] This factor is of particular significance because many countries permit vaccination exemptions based on religious grounds. There have also been headline-making outbreaks of vaccine preventable diseases in under-vaccinated religious communities around the world.[83] Various religious beliefs have been implicated as drivers of the vaccine hesitancy underlying such outbreaks. These include Christian concerns about vaccines utilising human cell lines derived from aborted foetuses in their production.[84] A minority of religious believers have also claimed that vaccines reduce people's dependence upon God and interfere with divine provenance, while others may forgo vaccines because of a dedication to faith healing and the idea that only God protects people from illness.[85] In relation to these ideas, Christian nationalism in the USA has been correlated with antivaccine sentiments.[86] Generally speaking, this worldview is associated with the premise that God, and not secular governments or science, is ultimately responsible for protecting the Christian nation of America.

Catholic and Protestant Christians, as well as members of the Church of Jesus Christ of Latter-Day Saints, have opposed human papilloma virus (HPV) vaccines because HPV is sexually transmitted. It has been claimed that allowing youth to receive the HPV vaccine tacitly encourages promiscuity.[87] Various Jewish and Islamic communities have resisted HPV vaccines on similar conservative religious grounds.[88] Conspiracies have also spread about vaccines being laced with ingredients to make Muslims infertile as part of an American plot to depopulate the Islamic world.[89] Worries have further been raised by some Muslims regarding misinformation about vaccines containing aborted foetal tissue, in addition to Islamic debates about whether certain vaccines are *halal* because they contain pork by-products.[90] In relation to vaccine ingredients, misinformation about COVID-19 vaccines containing traces of beef have also reportedly sparked immunisation uncertainties for Hindu adherents who are prohibited from eating cows.[91]

Along with the potential influence of religious beliefs, higher rates of religious participation and greater trust in religious leaders have been linked to vaccine hesitancy and misgivings abouts COVID-19 vaccines.[92] In the USA, greater religiosity was also associated with increased resistance to government-imposed COVID-19 restrictions, and lower intentions to get vaccinated against SARS-CoV-2.[93] Such observations, however, have not been universal, as other studies have failed to identify clear-cut links between religiosity with vaccine hesitancy.[94] In fact, an analysis of 147 countries reported that, contrary to most American findings, religious participation is "strongly positively correlated with country measures of confidence in the safety, importance, and effectiveness of vaccines."[95] Consequently, in many nations being religious is *more* likely to be associated with vaccine trust rather than hesitancy.

Together with religious affiliation and religious participation, there have been further connections identified between vaccine hesitancy and individuals who self-identify as being spiritual but not religious.[96] It has also been noted that antivaccination ideas "are often grounded in specific magical/spiritual health beliefs," and that such beliefs fit into "spiritual, not religious" categories rather than "traditional religious teachings."[97] Such magical/spiritual health beliefs have occasionally been connected with vaccine scepticism and positive attitudes toward complementary and alternative medicine, known as CAM.[98] Furthermore, elsewhere it has been identified that New Age spiritual beliefs and alternative health practices have together fused with conspiracy theories, which have been tied to online anti-COVID-19 lockdown and counter-vaccination messages.[99]

It seems then that connections between religiosity, religious affiliation, spirituality, trust in science and vaccine hesitancy are tricky to unravel, and they can vary according to country and cultural contexts.[100] It has also been questioned whether instances in which religion seems to be a barrier to vaccination truly have "a religious basis or not."[101] This is because direct associations between religion and vaccine refusal can be difficult to decipher. Immunisation doubts that at first appear to be tied to religious beliefs, for instance, may also be inextricably linked to local sociopolitical affiliations, cultural identities, and community networks, rather than the direct influence of religious doctrines themselves.[102] Aside from Christian Scientists, most major religions do not officially prohibit vaccines.[103] In fact, during the 19th century religious leaders represented some of the earliest public supporters of vaccination.[104] Other early responses to vaccination, however, described it as a "defiance to Heaven itself, even to the will of God."[105] These differing reactions reveal the complexities of religious perspectives on vaccination, which can sway vaccine intentions if an individual's local religious leaders or fellow community members express vaccine doubts.[106]

In brief, religious criticisms of vaccination can vary greatly from religion to religion. Even though most world religions support vaccination, and often consider it a moral obligation to be vaccinated, a range of religiously affiliated vaccine concerns may still foster counter-vaccine behaviours.[107] Be that as it may, research has found that the impact religion has on vaccination attitudes is frequently more dependent upon local social contexts, political affiliations and ideology, as well as networks associated with religious communities, rather than the direct influences of religious doctrines.[108]

6 Experiences

A Life history

An individual's past experiences with vaccinations can markedly influence future vaccine intentions. For instance, if an individual has previously had a negative encounter with a healthcare professional in relation to vaccines, or has experienced what they perceived to be adverse vaccine-induced side effects, they will be more reluctant to have their own children vaccinated.[109] Such experiences can heighten risk perceptions of vaccine dangers and increase uncertainties about vaccine safety.[110] Negative experiences involving poor interactions with health workers, including feeling coerced or scorned by doctors, as well as childhood memories of vaccine pain, are also shared between networks of relatives or friends and can influence vaccine decision-making.[111]

B Information needs

Some people also report experiencing greater needs for more information about vaccines. This includes individuals conveying that they have been given too little vaccination info from medical providers and received vaccine information that lacked enough detail to satisfy their questions.[112] Though it is important to remember that information deficits are frequently not the cause of vaccine hesitancy, there are those who feel that they require more detailed, and presumably unbiased, information as they make vaccination decisions. If they suspect that they are not receiving sufficiently detailed and impartial vaccine data from health professionals, they may be less inclined to vaccinate.[113]

7 Media

The significance of antivaccination media, as it relates to psychological factors affecting vaccine decision-making, is twofold. Firstly, as has been identified above, individuals often turn to online sources of information when they have questions about vaccination. People are predisposed to seek out online vaccination info for themselves, via such sources as websites, blogs and social media posts. Importantly, counter-immunisation online media can influence vaccination choices.[114] Secondly, such antivaccination media feature an assortment of arguments and persuasion attributes that can make their messages convincing to certain audiences.[115] These claims frequently tap into many of the key psychological factors listed above. For instance, counter-vaccine media often stresses the apparent risks of vaccinating, while referring to erroneous health intuitions.[116] It also questions the effectiveness of vaccines, refers to BigPharma vaccine conspiracies, while playing upon psychological reactance by claiming that mandatory vaccination policies take away our rights.[117]

Altogether, antivaccination media is important because some people actively seek it out, and such communications can also touch upon the core psychological factors influencing vaccine decision-making. To further unpack these factors, and to gain a deeper understanding about how persuasive counter-vaccination messages can impact audiences, it is necessary to move on and investigate the following three key topics:

1   The Cultural Cognition Thesis
2   Moral Foundations Theory
3   The Elaboration Likelihood Model of persuasion

The Cultural Cognition Thesis

There is a growing body of decision-making research labelled the *Cultural Cognition Thesis*, which was pioneered by Yale University's Dan Kahan and his research team. The aim of this work has been to uncover how ordinary people make risk calculations with regard to such topics as vaccines. In particular, Kahan's studies have investigated how individuals come to certain conclusions on such potentially contentious issues as climate change, disputes over gun control in the USA, and vaccinations.[118] What Kahan and his team discovered was that typically people tend to support whichever position on these issues best affirms the core values that define that individual's personal identities. Additionally, it has been found that people are inclined to stick to whatever position they already assumed to be true, rather than making decisions based on the objective facts and scientific data. With these findings in hand, Kahan developed the Cultural Cognition Thesis, which is centred around *identity-protective cognition*.

Identity-protective cognition has been described as the "tendency of people to fit their views to those of others with whom they share some important, self-identifying commitments."[119] Our links to the groups that we are affiliated with are incredibly strong, and frequently we shape our interpretation of science, including vaccines, to match up with the viewpoints of the people in those groups. This is because, accepting "beliefs at odds with those held by members of an identity-defining group" can be socially problematic, and can threaten the important community ties that we have with other group members.[120] A result of identity-protective cognition is that people are inclined to favour ideas that support the cultural worldviews that are maintained within the groups that they self-identify with.[121] Worldviews are the mental maps, cognitive frameworks, and cultural assumptions that a group shares to interpret, navigate and make sense of life. Worldviews shape and are shaped by our politics, our philosophies, our morals, beliefs, and values.

According to the Cultural Cognition Thesis, individuals make decisions about topics like vaccines that affirm their in-group identities and corroborate their loyalty to core group beliefs and values. As a result, people selectively accept or reject scientific facts in ways that validate their cultural worldviews. They agree with facts that they interpret to be compatible with their current beliefs, and they tend to be highly suspicious of any data that seems to conflict with the cultural values associated with their group networks.[122] As Dan Kahan has explained, people are "motivated, unconsciously, to conform to all manner of attitudes, including factual beliefs, to ones that are dominant within their self-defining reference groups."[123] Crucially, cultural cognition does not just influence what facts people accept or reject, but it also effects perceptions of other people's credibility and trustworthiness. Individuals tend to accept that an expert is trustworthy only if that specialist shares their own worldview.[124] For example, if a scientific expert on vaccines appears to not maintain the same cultural beliefs, or political values, as those held closely by a group of people, that audience is far less likely to accept the scientific expert's opinion, even though that opinion is based on empirical evidence and years of scientific training.[125]

What is insightful about Cultural Cognition Thesis research is that it has involved measuring and mapping the worldviews that so strongly influence people's acceptance or rejection of science. This has been achieved by using

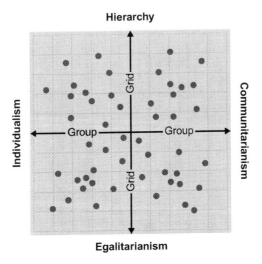

Figure 2.2 Cultural Cognition Map[126]

the two intersecting scales featured in Figure 2.2, and then plotting where people lie on the resulting graph. The scale running from top to bottom is described as the *Grid* scale, and it has attributes of "Hierarchy" at the top and "Egalitarianism" at the bottom. People who have greater respect for authority and believe that hierarchies and power differences are a natural, healthy part of societies would score toward the top of this scale. These people might advocate for traditional values and roles, and they would support societies based on stratified ranks distributed according to privilege, different abilities, gender, or age. They might agree with the statement, "We have gone too far in pushing equal rights in this country."[127] Others who believe that goods and services, as well as jobs and public offices should be equally open and available to everyone, rather than according to ranks or social hierarchies, would fall towards Egalitarianism at the bottom. These individuals would be more likely to agree with the statement, "Our society would be better off if the distribution of wealth was more equal."[128]

The scale extending from left to right is the *Group* scale, and it has "Individualism" on the left, and "Communitarianism" on the right. Someone who has individualistic values, who appreciates personal initiative, without other people or government meddling in their affairs, would fall toward the left side of the scale. These individuals might contend that people should competitively fend for themselves without help from others. Such people would probably agree with the statement, "Society works best when it lets individuals take responsibility for their own lives without telling them what to do."[129] Alternatively, a person who has cultural values focussed on people helping each other in society would map onto the Communitarianism side of the scale. Such an individual would be more likely to agree with the statement, "It's society's responsibility to make sure everyone's basic needs are met."[130]

Research has further demonstrated that there are often correlations between where people fall on the Grid-Group scales and their views on science. For instance, hierarchical-individualists (top-left) tend to value free enterprise and business success, while believing that society should not be overregulated by governments. Hierarchical-individualists also tend to be the most sceptical of climate change science, because it brings with it the need for environmental guidelines for corporations that may hinder commerce. Individuals who are egalitarian-communitarian (bottom-right) are polarised the other way.[131] Remarkably, when people's scientific knowledge increases, they can actually become more divided on issues such as climate change or vaccines according to their worldview associations and cultural identity affiliations. Plus, in line with supposition that the Information Deficit Model is intrinsically flawed, it has been revealed that giving people facts can actually reinforce persistent beliefs rather than change minds.[132]

Research into the influences of cultural orientations on vaccine attitudes appear to compliment the Cultural Cognition Thesis. For instance, studies have identified certain cultural predictors of vaccine hesitancy. People expressing collectivist cultural attitudes, especially those who believe in equality, may be more inclined to get vaccinated.[133] This outlook is relatively analogous to communitarian-egalitarianism on the Cultural Cognition Map. With a collectivist cultural mindset, communal goals are given priority, and individual ambitions are put second to the needs of a community.[134] As a result, vaccination is perceived to be a collective obligation that protects others through herd immunity. This overrides personal wishes or immunisation reluctance, particularly for collectivists who value equality. On the other hand, people who have individualist cultural orientations, who also express hierarchical views of society, including accepting inequalities as natural, tend to be more vaccine hesitant.[135] This position is more akin to hierarchical-individualism on the Cultural Cognition Map. With individualism, personal needs and rights are given priority over communal goals.[136]

Reports on cultural orientations and vaccine attitudes propose that pro-vaccination messages should be customised to reach the hesitant hierarchical individualists (Chapter 6).[137] More effective messages will line up with people's cultural outlooks and values. Likewise, it has been found that people lean towards accepting vaccine information from experts who share their own worldview values, but they are prone to resist vaccine arguments from an expert whose values they oppose.[138] People's worldviews play a fundamental role in whether they accept scientific evidence from experts or not. The degree to which vaccination authorities seem to be trusted hinges upon how well the cultural values of such experts appear to align with those of the audience, and people's interpretations of the same scientific facts is strongly influenced by worldview biases. This is why the Cultural Cognition Thesis is perhaps one of the most vital concepts to understand about vaccine decision-making.

Moral Foundations Theory

In connection with the many factors that can influence how people make vaccination decisions, it is also important to discuss the impact of moral values, and more specifically, the *Moral Foundations Theory*. Developed by Jonathan Haidt and Jesse Graham, this psychological theory addresses how people's emotionally driven moral intuitions can frequently guide decision-making. It identifies several key psychological foundations of morality that seem to produce quick and automatic emotional reactions. These moral foundations are thought to be instinctive, operating at the gut-level, and they often guide how people make judgements in everyday life.[139] Haidt and Graham have identified six central foundations, which are described as: care/harm, fairness/cheating, loyalty/betrayal, authority/subversion, sanctity/degradation, and liberty/oppression (Table 2.1).[140]

It should be noted that the degree to which different communities emphasise or minimise their focus on each of these foundations varies across

Table 2.1 Moral foundations

1. Care/harm
This foundation encompasses people's concern for the wellbeing of others. The intuition involves our natural impulses to protect our own children and other people from harm.[141] It includes upholding such virtues as compassion, kindness, and caring for the vulnerable.
2. Fairness/cheating
The fairness/cheating dimension relates to treating people fairly, maintaining justice, and defending the rights of citizens. It can also include protecting personal autonomy. This foundation is related to the idea that "people should be rewarded in proportion to what they contribute," and be reciprocally punished for taking advantage of others.[142]
3. Loyalty/betrayal
This moral intuition involves dedication to group membership, the distrust of non-group individuals and traitors, as well as respecting self-sacrifice for one's community. These drives are integrated into patriotic impulses. The foundation helps to contribute to "effective tribalism and success in inter-group competition."[143]
4. Authority/subversion
This emotional dimension includes instinctive respect for hierarchy, obedience to legitimate authority, duty, awe, and admiration for those in power, as well as maintaining respect for traditions. The authority/subversion foundation incorporates the "demand that respect be shown to parents, teachers, and others in positions of authority."[144] At the heart of this foundation is the desire to protect the perceived order of things and avoid chaos.
5. Sanctity/degradation
The sanctity/degradation foundation exemplifies the psychology of disgust and prevention of contamination. This is connected with desires to avoid diseases and parasites. The intuition is also linked to concepts of religious sacredness, in which some ideas or objects are treated as having inviolable value. Sanctity/degradation "makes it easy for us to regard some things as 'untouchable,' both in a bad way (because something is so dirty or polluted we want to stay away) and in a good way (because something is so hallowed, so sacred, that we want to protect it from desecration)."[145]
6. Liberty/oppression
The sixth dimension is associated with negative emotional reactions and resentment towards dominant people and institutions, as well as our responses to the restriction of civil liberties. Related to psychological reactance (p. 40), this foundation triggers people's dislike of bullies and the protection of freedoms, which can motivate people to unite against oppressors.[146]

cultures and subcultures.[147] With these considerations in mind, Moral Foundation Theory still proves useful for some decision-making research, as it has drawn attention to the way that emotion-driven, instinctive moral sensitivities can influence our attitudes and behaviours.[148] Studies have found that political orientation, including liberal or conservative political leanings in the USA, as well as whether individuals support vaccine science, appear to be somewhat associated with these emotionally laden intuitions.[149] Citizens ascribing to liberal political principles generally hold chiefly to only the foundations of care/harm and fairness/cheating, while conservatives rely upon a more evenly distributed blend of each foundation.[150] As a result, for conservative-minded individuals, compassion and fairness constitute only one-third of their moral profiles, which are counterbalanced by the remaining foundations.[151]

Attitudes toward scientific theories seem moderately related to the influences of certain moral foundations. One study, for instance, analysed the outcomes of morally framing pro-environmental messages for American conservatives, who generally articulate less concern for environmental crises, including anthropogenic climate change, than their politically liberal counterparts.[152] The researchers took into account the tendencies of conservative leaning individuals to stress the loyalty/betrayal, authority/subversion, sanctity/degradation, and liberty/oppression foundations, which extend beyond the care/harm and fairness/cheating intuitions that political progressives usually focus on. They then communicated pro-environmental messages to conservative audiences, which framed eco-protection as a matter of American patriotism, and submitting to legitimate authority, as well as defending the purity of nature. The result was that, in comparison to non-moral appeals, conservative leaning individuals significantly shifted their attitudes in support of pro-environmental activity.

Regarding vaccinations, some research suggests that people with high levels of vaccine hesitancy have beliefs strongly tied to the sanctity/degradation foundation. This is because they perceive vaccines to be biological purity "violations (for example, vaccines contain poisons and toxins, while diseases like measles are natural)."[153] Fervent vaccine hesitancy also seems related to a heightened sense of liberty/oppression, since people with hesitations tend to view compulsory vaccination policies as violations of their civil liberties, and unreasonable government control.[154] People who are undecided or opposed to vaccines, also can express lower levels of respect for those in positions of authority.[155]

All in all, the Moral Foundations Theory provides an additional perspective on vaccination decision-making that connects with other observations about vaccine hesitancy. For instance, issues pertaining to the sanctity/degradation foundation seem to overlap with reports that fear, and disgust can influence vaccine choices. Concerns related to the fairness/cheating foundation also appear to coincide with issues of distrust and psychological reactance. Likewise, it seems that pro-science messages which appeal to an audience's moral intuitions can be more persuasive. Finally, the Moral Foundations Theory again highlights the fundamental point that people make decisions based on numerous social and psychological influences, such as instinctive moral intuitions, rather than just on facts. This leads us to one last important concept to consider regarding how people tend to make decisions: *The Elaboration Likelihood Model* of persuasion. By learning about this model, it is possible to gain an added understanding regarding how people may respond to persuasive media about vaccines.

The Elaboration Likelihood Model of persuasion

For decades, researchers have been fascinated with mass media and its potential for persuasion.[156] Analysts have reported on the impacts of news broadcasts and political campaigns on public opinion, and examined how violence in media can affect people, as well as the outcomes of healthcare communications in influencing audiences.[157] In addition to such research, it is also clear that staggering amounts of money are being spent worldwide on consumer advertising, political communication campaigns, and even military mass persuasion operations.[158] It should be asked whether all of this capital would be devoted to these efforts if there were not at least some discernible results. Moreover, these sums are being spent even though most individuals are inclined to say that they are resistant to the effects of persuasive media. This tendency, known as the *third-person effect*, results from the feeling that others are more gullible than us.[159] This effect is also related to what has been described as the *Media Manipulation Denial Syndrome*. This is a widespread tendency for people to not admit that they are personally affected by media effects. Nevertheless, though individuals do not generally think that they are personally affected by media persuasion, research demonstrates that these same individuals are in fact swayed by media influences.[160]

If evidence exists that media persuasion can influence publics, how exactly does media persuasion work? This question is important for vaccine hesitancy and decision-making because media for-and-against vaccinating may be helping to shape public opinion around the world today. To answer this query it is helpful to turn to persuasion research, and the Elaboration Likelihood Model of persuasion (ELM). The ELM is one of the most robust and enduring persuasion theories, which was developed by Richard E. Petty and John T. Cacioppo.[162] It suggests that there are two major avenues of persuasion that result from being exposed to communications, including media that may support or attack vaccines. These two avenues are labelled the *central* and *peripheral* routes of persuasion.[163] The central route involves attitude change through an individual's careful analysis of a persuasive message. This is described as high elaboration, which involves using a significant amount of mental effort to carefully examine the quality and logic of a message's arguments. For high elaboration to occur, a person must have both the motivation and the ability to methodically study a communication's claims. Motivation and processing ability increase the likelihood of elaboration, which will lead to either favourable or unfavourable responses to a message's persuasive claims. When central route thinking occurs, and elaboration likelihood is high, a person's response will generally be shaped by the quality of a persuasive message's arguments and its data.[164]

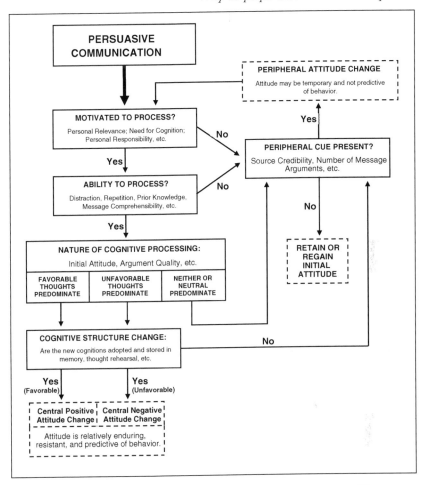

Figure 2.3 A schematic depiction of the Elaboration Likelihood Model[161]

The peripheral route, on the other hand, consists of low elaboration. This occurs when someone simply lacks the time, or the motivation, or the ability to thoroughly investigate and process a persuasive message's claims. The low elaboration avenue involves comparatively little cognitive exertion. What is important about it is that, instead of systematically dissecting a persuasive communication, low elaboration involves depending upon "mental shortcuts," or "cues," found in a message to come to a conclusion about its claims.[165] These cues have been described as "stimuli in the persuasion context that can affect attitudes without necessitating processing of the message arguments."[166] Such cues can include a messenger's perceived credibility (Chapter 3).

Even though most people want to hold correct attitudes, insufficient education about communicated topics, or a lack of time or motivation needed to scrutinise claims, combined with the immense amount of persuasive messages that individuals confront on a daily basis, means that people frequently engage in peripheral route persuasion.[167] Also, if central cognitive processing results in neither a positive nor a negative reaction, or if there is no clear change in that person's views, peripheral processing may still occur. According to the Elaboration Likelihood Model, central route persuasion leads to enduring attitude change, that is more predicative of behaviour than persuasion resulting from the peripheral route.[168] However, both routes still prove to be crucial paths of persuasion, and empirical research has helped to demonstrate the effectiveness of peripheral route attitude formation.[169]

From the ELM to counter-vaccine persuasion and myths

Through its findings, the Elaboration Likelihood Model has provided key insights into how persuasion operates. This is especially valuable because widespread messages, including antivaccination claims and counter-vaccine social media posts, can be an important element in vaccine decision-making. As this book will investigate in greater detail moving forward, antivaccination communications often contain several persuasive cues that have been found to influence audiences. The next chapter will begin unpacking such persuasion elements, as well as several vaccination myths commonly exhibited in counter-vaccine messages. Even though committed vaccine deniers and vaccine hesitant individuals from across the globe do not belong to a single homogenous group, antivaccination arguments and persuasion strategies are often remarkably similar. As Chapter 3 will reveal, these similarities are expressed in three common themes of antivaccination media, which can be described as: *Distrust, Confidence,* and *Danger.*

Notes

1   Chiara Cadeddu et al., "Beliefs Towards Vaccination and Trust in the Scientific Community in Italy," *Vaccine* 38, no. 42 (2020); Catherine Helps et al., "Understanding Non-Vaccinating Parents' Views to Inform and Improve Clinical Encounters: A Qualitative Study in an Australian Community," *BMJ* 9, no. 5 (2019); Matt Motta et al., "Identifying the Prevalence, Correlates, and Policy Consequences of Anti-Vaccine Social Identity," *Politics, Groups & Identities* ahead-of-print, no. ahead-of-print (2021); Kim A. G. J. Romijnders et al., "A Deliberate Choice? Exploring Factors Related to Informed Decision-Making About Childhood Vaccination among Acceptors, Refusers, and Partial Acceptors," *Vaccine* 37, no. 37 (2019).
2   Aida Bianco et al., "Parent Perspectives on Childhood Vaccination: How to Deal with Vaccine Hesitancy and Refusal?," *Vaccine* no. 7; Stefania Dzieciolowska et al., "Covid-19 Vaccine Acceptance, Hesitancy, and Refusal among Canadian Healthcare Workers: A Multicenter Survey," *American Journal of Infection Control* 49, no. 9 (2021); T. Rozbroj, A. Lyons, and J. Lucke, "Vaccine-Hesitant and Vaccine-Refusing Parents' Reflections on the Way

Parenthood Changed Their Attitudes to Vaccination," *Journal of Community Health* 45, no. 1 (2020).

3 Ho P. Huynh and Amy R. Senger, "A Little Shot of Humility: Intellectual Humility Predicts Vaccination Attitudes and Intention to Vaccinate against Covid-19," *Journal of the American Pharmacists Association* 51, no. 4 (2021); Amy R. Senger and Ho P. Huynh, "Intellectual Humility's Association with Vaccine Attitudes and Intentions," *Psychology, Health & Medicine* 26, no. 9 (2021); Matthew Motta, Timothy Callaghan, and Steven Sylvester, "Knowing Less but Presuming More: Dunning-Kruger Effects and the Endorsement of Anti-Vaccine Policy Attitudes," *Social Science & Medicine* 211 (2018).

4 Daniel Jolley and Karen M. Douglas, "The Effects of Anti-Vaccine Conspiracy Theories on Vaccination Intentions," *PLoS One* 9, no. 2 (2014); Helena Tomljenovic, Andreja Bubic, and Nikola Erceg, "It Just Doesn't Feel Right – the Relevance of Emotions and Intuition for Parental Vaccine Conspiracy Beliefs and Vaccination Uptake," *Psychology & Health* 35, no. 5 (2020).

5 Lindsay Wilson et al., "Barriers to Immunization among Newcomers: A Systematic Review," *Vaccine* 36, no. 8 (2018); Litjen Tan, "A Review of the Key Factors to Improve Adult Immunization Coverage Rates: What Can the Clinician Do?," *Vaccine* no. 36.

6 Helps et al., "Understanding Non-Vaccinating Parents' Views to Inform and Improve Clinical Encounters: A Qualitative Study in an Australian Community," 3.

7 Astrid Austvoll-Dahlgren and Sølvi Helseth, "What Informs Parents' Decision-Making About Childhood Vaccinations?," *Journal of Advanced Nursing* 66, no. 11 (2010).

8 Anne M. Walsh et al., "Use of Online Health Information to Manage Children's Health Care: A Prospective Study Investigating Parental Decisions," *BMC Health Services Research* 15, no. 1 (2015); Maria Chow et al., "Parental Attitudes, Beliefs, Behaviours and Concerns Towards Childhood Vaccinations in Australia: A National Online Survey," *Australian Family Physician* 46, no. 3 (2017); Matthew Z. Dudley et al., "Words Matter: Vaccine Hesitancy, Vaccine Demand, Vaccine Confidence, Herd Immunity and Mandatory Vaccination," *Vaccine* 38, no. 4 (2020); Neha Puri et al., "Social Media and Vaccine Hesitancy: New Updates for the Era of COVID-19 and Globalized Infectious Diseases," *Hum Vaccin Immunother* 16, no. 11 (2020).

9 Courtney Babaoff and Jennifer P. D'Auria, "Googling for Information About Alternative Vaccination Schedules," *Journal of Pediatric Health Care* 29, no. 4 (2015); Elisa J. Sobo et al., "Information Curation among Vaccine Cautious Parents: Web 2.0, Pinterest Thinking, and Pediatric Vaccination Choice," *Medical Anthropology* 35, no. 6 (2016); M. S. Smailbegovic, G. J. Laing, and H. Bedford, "Why Do Parents Decide against Immunization? The Effect of Health Beliefs and Health Professionals," *Child: Care, Health and Development* 29, no. 4 (2003).

10 Craig Smith, Claire Duffy, and Michelle Kirszner, *Research to Identify Immunisation Information Needs: Qualitative Research Report* (Crows Nest: Department of Health, 2016), 74.

11 Anna Kata, "A Postmodern Pandora's Box: Anti-Vaccination Misinformation on the Internet," *Vaccine* 28, no. 7 (2010); Cornelia Betsch and Katharina Sachse, "Dr. Jekyll or Mr. Hyde? (How) the Internet Influences Vaccination Decisions: Recent Evidence and Tentative Guidelines for Online Vaccine Communication," *Vaccine* 30, no. 25 (2012); Mohan J. Dutta-Bergman, "Primary Sources of Health Information: Comparisons in the Domain of Health Attitudes, Health Cognitions, and Health Behaviors," *Health Communication* 16, no. 3 (2004); Melissa Fryer, "The Influence of the Internet of Children's

Vaccination: Applying Intercultural Theories to Analyze Parental Decision-Making," *Journal of Media Critiques* 2, no. 8 (2016); Robert M. Wolfe, Lisa K. Sharp, and Martin S. Lipsky, "Content and Design Attributes of Antivaccination Web Sites," *JAMA* 287, no. 24 (2002).

12 B. Narayan and M. Preljevic, "An Information Behaviour Approach to Conspiracy Theories: Listening in on Voices from within the Vaccination Debate," *Information Research* 22, no. 1 (2017).

13 Koji Wada and Derek R. Smith, "Mistrust Surrounding Vaccination Recommendations by the Japanese Government: Results from a National Survey of Working-Age Individuals Health Behavior, Health Promotion and Society," *BMC Public Health* 15, no. 1 (2015); Yunmi Chung et al., "Influences on Immunization Decision-Making among US Parents of Young Children," *Maternal and Child Health Journal* 21, no. 12 (2017); Jamie Murphy et al., "Psychological Characteristics Associated with COVID-19 Vaccine Hesitancy and Resistance in Ireland and the United Kingdom," *Nature Communications* 12, no. 1 (2021).

14 Jordan Lee Tustin et al., "Internet Exposure Associated with Canadian Parents' Perception of Risk on Childhood Immunization: Cross-Sectional Study," *JMIR Public Health and Surveillance* 4, no. 1 (2018); Francesco Pierri et al., "Online Misinformation Is Linked to Early COVID-19 Vaccination Hesitancy and Refusal," *Scientific Reports* 12, no. 1 (2022); Amanda Hudson and William J. Montelpare, "Predictors of Vaccine Hesitancy: Implications for COVID-19 Public Health Messaging," *International Journal of Environmental Research and Public Health* 18, no. 15 (2021).

15 Matteo Cinelli et al., "The COVID-19 Social Media Infodemic," *Scientific Reports* 10, no. 1 (2020); Yuxi Wang et al., "Systematic Literature Review on the Spread of Health-Related Misinformation on Social Media," *Social Science & Medicine* 240 (2019).

16 Nadia Arif et al., "Fake News or Weak Science? Visibility and Characterization of Antivaccine Webpages Returned by Google in Different Languages and Countries," *Frontiers in Immunology* 9 (2018).

17 Kata, "A Postmodern Pandora's Box: Anti-Vaccination Misinformation on the Internet," 36–41; Puri et al., "Social Media and Vaccine Hesitancy: New Updates for the Era of COVID-19 and Globalized Infectious Diseases."; Sahrish Ekram et al., "Content and Commentary: HPV Vaccine and Youtube," *Journal of Pediatric and Adolescent Gynecology* 32, no. 2 (2019); Lisa Singh et al., "A First Look at COVID-19 Information and Misinformation Sharing on Twitter," *arXiv* 2003, no. 13907 (2020).

18 Federico Germani and Nikola Biller-Andorno, "The Anti-Vaccination Infodemic on Social Media: A Behavioral Analysis," *PLoS One* 16, no. 3 (2021).

19 Kai-Cheng Yang et al., "The COVID-19 Infodemic: Twitter Versus Facebook," *Big Data & Society* 8, no. 1 (2021).

20 Gianluca Nogara et al., "The Disinformation Dozen: An Exploratory Analysis of Covid-19 Disinformation Proliferation on Twitter" (paper presented at the 14th ACM Web Science Conference, New York, 2022).

21 Narayan and Preljevic, "An Information Behaviour Approach to Conspiracy Theories: Listening in on Voices from within the Vaccination Debate."; Wolfe, Sharp, and Lipsky, "Content and Design Attributes of Antivaccination Web Sites."; Betsch and Sachse, "Dr. Jekyll or Mr. Hyde."; Fryer, "The Influence of the Internet of Children's Vaccination: Applying Intercultural Theories to Analyze Parental Decision-Making."; Sabrina Heike Kessler and Arne Freya Zillich, "Searching Online for Information About Vaccination: Assessing the Influence of User-Specific Cognitive Factors Using Eye-Tracking," *Health Communication* 20 (2018).

22 Jinxuan Ma and Lynne Stahl, "A Multimodal Critical Discourse Analysis of Anti-Vaccination Information on Facebook," *Library and Information Science Research* 39, no. 4 (2017): 304; Thomas Aechtner, "Improving Evolution Advocacy: Translating Vaccine Interventions to the Evolution Wars," *Zygon* 55, no. 1 (2020).

23 Timothy Caulfield, Alessandro R. Marcon, and Blake Murdoch, "Injecting Doubt: Responding to the Naturopathic Anti-Vaccination Rhetoric," *Journal of Law and the Biosciences* 4, no. 2 (2017); Graham N. Dixon and Christopher E. Clarke, "Heightening Uncertainty around Certain Science: Media Coverage, False Balance, and the Autism-Vaccine Controversy," *Science Communication* 35, no. 3 (2013); Cornelia Betsch, "Innovations in Communication: The Internet and the Psychology of Vaccination Decisions," *Eurosurveillance* 16, no. 17 (2011); Cornelia Betsch et al., "The Influence of Vaccine-Critical Websites on Perceiving Vaccination Risks," *Journal of Health Psychology* 15, no. 3 (2010).

24 Caulfield, Marcon, and Murdoch, "Injecting Doubt: Responding to the Naturopathic Anti-Vaccination Rhetoric," 11.

25 Ana Lucía Schmidt et al., "Polarization of the Vaccination Debate on Facebook," *Vaccine* 36, no. 25 (2018); Marianna Zummo, "A Linguistic Analysis of the Online Debate on Vaccines and Use of Fora as Information Stations and Confirmation Niche," *International Journal of Society, Culture & Language* 5, no. 1 (2017); Jeanette B. Ruiz and Robert A. Bell, "Understanding Vaccination Resistance: Vaccine Search Term Selection Bias and the Valence of Retrieved Information," *Vaccine* 32, no. 44 (2014).

26 Anthony Nadler, Matthew Crain, and Joan Donovan, *Weaponizing the Digital Influence Machine: The Political Perils of Online Ad Tech* (New York: Data & Society Research Institute, 2018), 4–8.

27 Marcel Salathé and Shashank Khandelwal, "Assessing Vaccination Sentiments with Online Social Media: Implications for Infectious Disease Dynamics and Control," *PLoS Computational Biology* 7, no. 10 (2011).

28 Noel T. Brewer et al., "Increasing Vaccination: Putting Psychological Science into Action," *Psychological Science in the Public Interest* 18, no. 3 (2017): 168.

29 P. Sol Hart and Erik C. Nisbet, "Boomerang Effects in Science Communication: How Motivated Reasoning and Identity Cues Amplify Opinion Polarization About Climate Mitigation Policies," *Communication Research* 39, no. 6 (2012).

30 Norbert Schwarz et al., "Metacognitive Experiences and the Intricacies of Setting People Straight: Implications for Debiasing and Public Information Campaigns," *Advances in Experimental Social Psychology* 39 (2007): 127–28.

31 Catherine C. McClure, Jessica R. Cataldi, and Sean T. O'Leary, "Vaccine Hesitancy: Where We Are and Where We Are Going," *Clinical Therapeutics* 39, no. 8 (2017); Heidi J. Larson et al., "Addressing the Vaccine Confidence Gap," *Lancet* 378, no. 9790 (2011); Jacqueline R. Meszaros et al., "Cognitive Processes and the Decisions of Some Parents to Forego Pertussis Vaccination for Their Children," *Journal of Clinical Epidemiology* 49, no. 6 (1996).

32 Brendan Nyhan and Jason Reifler, "Does Correcting Myths About the Flu Vaccine Work? An Experimental Evaluation of the Effects of Corrective Information," *Vaccine* 33, no. 3 (2015); Dan Kahan et al., "Motivated Numeracy and Enlightened Self-Government," *Behavioural Public Policy* 1, no. 1 (2017): 78–79; Angus Thomson, Karis Robinson, and Gaëlle Vallée-Tourangeau, "The 5as: A Practical Taxonomy for the Determinants of Vaccine Uptake," *Vaccine* 34, no. 8 (2016): 1022.

33 Dan Kahan et al., "Geoengineering and Climate Change Polarization," *The ANNALS of the American Academy of Political and Social Science* 658, no. 1 (2015).

34 Eve Dubé et al., "Vaccine Hesitancy: An Overview," *Human Vaccines & Immunotherapeutics* 9, no. 8 (2013): 1768.

35 Joseph O. Baker, "Acceptance of Evolution and Support for Teaching Creationism in Public Schools: The Conditional Impact of Educational Attainment," *Journal for the Scientific Study of Religion* 52, no. 1 (2013): 225–26.

36 McClure, Cataldi, and O'Leary, "Vaccine Hesitancy: Where We Are and Where We Are Going," 1554.

37 Stephan Lewandowsky and Klaus Oberauer, "Motivated Rejection of Science," *Current Directions in Psychological Science* 25, no. 4 (2016): 218.

38 Susanna Priest, "Critical Science Literacy: Making Sense of Science," in *Communicating Climate Change: The Path Forward*, ed. Susanna Priest (London: Palgrave Macmillan, 2016).

39 Tara C. Smith, "Vaccine Rejection and Hesitancy: A Review and Call to Action," *Open Forum Infectious Diseases* 4, no. 3 (2017).

40 Emily K. Brunson, "How Parents Make Decisions About Their Children's Vaccinations," *Vaccine* 31, no. 46 (2013); A. Lynne Sturm, M. Rose Mays, and D. Gregory Zimet, "Parental Beliefs and Decision Making About Child and Adolescent Immunization: From Polio to Sexually Transmitted Infections," *Journal of Developmental & Behavioral Pediatrics* 26, no. 6 (2005); Morgan Melanie et al., "Identifying Relevant Anti-Science Perceptions to Improve Science-Based Communication: The Negative Perceptions of Science Scale," *Social Sciences* 7, no. 4 (2018); Pieter Streefland, A. M. R. Chowdhury, and Pilar Ramos-Jimenez, "Patterns of Vaccination Acceptance," *Social Science & Medicine* 49, no. 12 (1999); Brendan Nyhan, Jason Reifler, and Sean Richey, "The Role of Social Networks in Influenza Vaccine Attitudes and Intentions among College Students in the Southeastern United States," *Journal of Adolescent Health* 51, no. 3 (2012); Matthew Browne, "Epistemic Divides and Ontological Confusions: The Psychology of Vaccine Scepticism," *Human Vaccines & Immunotherapeutics* (2018).

41 Smailbegovic, Laing, and Bedford, "Why Do Parents Decide against Immunization? The Effect of Health Beliefs and Health Professionals," 307.

42 Allison Kempe et al., "Prevalence of Parental Concerns About Childhood Vaccines: The Experience of Primary Care Physicians," *American Journal of Preventive Medicine* 40, no. 5 (2011).

43 Ibid., 4807; Daniel Freeman et al., "Injection Fears and COVID-19 Vaccine Hesitancy," *Psychological Medicine* (2021).

44 Allison Kennedy, Michelle Basket, and Kristine Sheedy, "Vaccine Attitudes, Concerns, and Information Sources Reported by Parents of Young Children: Results from the 2009 Healthstyles Survey," *Pediatrics* 127 suppl 1, no. 1 (2011).

45 Russ Clay, "The Behavioral Immune System and Attitudes About Vaccines: Contamination Aversion Predicts More Negative Vaccine Attitudes," *Social Psychological and Personality Science* 8, no. 2 (2017).

46 Matthew J. Hornsey, Emily A. Harris, and Kelly S. Fielding, "The Psychological Roots of Anti-Vaccination Attitudes: A 24-Nation Investigation," *Health Psychology* 37, no. 4 (2018).

47 Jennifer A. Reich, "Of Natural Bodies and Antibodies: Parents' Vaccine Refusal and the Dichotomies of Natural and Artificial," *Social Science & Medicine* 157 (2016).

48 Richard Reading, "Children's Health and the Social Theory of Risk: Insights from the British Measles, Mumps and Rubella (MMR) Controversy," *Child: Care, Health and Development* 33, no. 6 (2007); T. G. W. Paulussen et al., "Determinants of Dutch Parents' Decisions to Vaccinate Their Child," *Vaccine* 24, no. 5 (2006).

49 Mike Poltorak et al., "'MMR Talk' and Vaccination Choices: An Ethnographic Study in Brighton," *Social Science & Medicine* 61, no. 3 (2005): 716.

50 Dubé et al., "Vaccine Hesitancy: An Overview," 1769.

51 Katrina F. Brown et al., "UK Parents' Decision-Making About Measles–Mumps–Rubella (MMR) Vaccine 10 Years after the MMR-Autism Controversy: A Qualitative Analysis," *Vaccine* 30, no. 10 (2012); Benjamin Gardner et al., "Beliefs Underlying UK Parents' Views Towards MMR Promotion Interventions: A Qualitative Study," *Psychology, Health & Medicine* 15, no. 2 (2010); Noel T. Brewer et al., "Meta-Analysis of the Relationship between Risk Perception and Health Behavior: The Example of Vaccination," *Health Psychology* 26, no. 2 (2007).

52 Diane Bolton-Maggs et al., "Perceptions of Mumps and MMR Vaccination among University Students in England: An Online Survey," *Vaccine* 30, no. 34 (2012); Gardner et al., "Beliefs Underlying UK Parents' Views Towards MMR Promotion Interventions: A Qualitative Study."

53 Melissa Leach and James Fairhead, *Vaccine Anxieties: Global Science, Child Health, and Society* (London: Earthscan, 2007), 22.

54 Poltorak et al., "'MMR Talk' and Vaccination Choices: An Ethnographic Study in Brighton," 715–16.

55 Shona Hilton, Mark Petticrew, and Kate Hunt, "'Combined Vaccines Are Like a Sudden Onslaught to the Body's Immune System': Parental Concerns About Vaccine 'Overload' and 'Immune-Vulnerability'," *Vaccine* 24, no. 20 (2006): 4322.

56 Kata, "A Postmodern Pandora's Box: Anti-Vaccination Misinformation on the Internet," 1711–12.

57 Patrick Davies, Simon Chapman, and Julie Leask, "Antivaccination Activists on the World Wide Web," *Archives of Disease in Childhood* 87, no. 1 (2002): 24; Julie-Anne Leask and Simon Chapman, "'An Attempt to Swindle Nature': Press Anti-Immunisation Reportage 1993–1997," *Australian and New Zealand Journal of Public Health* 22, no. 1 (1998): 19–20.

58 Robert M. Wolfe and Lisa K. Sharp, "Anti-Vaccinationists Past and Present," *BMJ* 325, no. 7361 (2002).

59 Robert M. Wolfe, "Vaccine Safety Activists on the Internet," *Expert Review of Vaccines* 1, no. 3 (2002): 250.

60 Pru Hobson-West, "'Trusting Blindly Can Be the Biggest Risk of All': Organised Resistance to Childhood Vaccination in the UK," *Sociology of Health & Illness* 29, no. 2 (2007); Streefland, Chowdhury, and Ramos-Jimenez, "Patterns of Vaccination Acceptance."; Jeffrey V. Lazarus et al., "A Survey of COVID-19 Vaccine Acceptance across 23 Countries in 2022," *Nature Medicine* (2023).

61 Andrea L. Benin et al., "Qualitative Analysis of Mothers' Decision-Making About Vaccines for Infants: The Importance of Trust," *Pediatrics* 117, no. 5 (2006).

62 Gary L. Freed et al., "Sources and Perceived Credibility of Vaccine-Safety Information for Parents," *Pediatrics* 127 suppl 1, no. 1 (2011); B. G. Gellin, E. W. Maibach, and E. K. Marcuse, "Do Parents Understand Immunizations? A National Telephone Survey," *Pediatrics* 106, no. 5 (2000); Romijnders et al., "A Deliberate Choice? Exploring Factors Related to Informed Decision-Making About Childhood Vaccination among Acceptors, Refusers, and Partial Acceptors."

63 Gardner et al., "Beliefs Underlying UK Parents' Views Towards MMR Promotion Interventions: A Qualitative Study."

64 Sachiko Ozawa and Meghan L Stack, "Public Trust and Vaccine Acceptance—International Perspectives," *Human Vaccines & Immunotherapeutics* 9, no. 8 (2013): 1777.

65 Cass R. Sunstein and Adrian Vermeule, "Conspiracy Theories: Causes and Cures," *Journal of Political Philosophy* 17, no. 2 (2009): 205.

66 L. F. Vernon, "Is Vaccine Dissent Based on Science?," *Health Education and Care* 2, no. 4 (2017); Jacob Heller, "Trust in Institutions, Science and Self – the Case of Vaccines," *Narrative Inquiry in Bioethics* 6, no. 3 (2016); Thomas Aechtner, "Distrust, Danger, and Confidence: A Content Analysis of the Australian Vaccination-Risks Network Blog," *Public Understanding of Science* (2020).

67 Jolley and Douglas, "The Effects of Anti-Vaccine Conspiracy Theories on Vaccination Intentions."

68 Hornsey, Harris, and Fielding, "The Psychological Roots of Anti-Vaccination Attitudes: A 24-Nation Investigation."; Jolley and Douglas, "The Effects of Anti-Vaccine Conspiracy Theories on Vaccination Intentions."; Stephan Lewandowsky, Gilles E. Gignac, and Klaus Oberauer, "The Role of Conspiracist Ideation and Worldviews in Predicting Rejection of Science," *PLoS One* 8, no. 10 (2013); Lisset Martinez-Berman, Lynn McCutcheon, and Ho P. Huynh, "Is the Worship of Celebrities Associated with Resistance to Vaccinations? Relationships between Celebrity Admiration, Anti-Vaccination Attitudes, and Beliefs in Conspiracy," *Psychology, Health & Medicine* 26, no. 9 (2021); Naomi Smith and Tim Graham, "Mapping the Anti-Vaccination Movement on Facebook," *Information, Communication & Society* 22, no. 9 (2019); Tomljenovic, Bubic, and Erceg, "It Just Doesn't Feel Right – the Relevance of Emotions and Intuition for Parental Vaccine Conspiracy Beliefs and Vaccination Uptake."

69 Zachary J. Goldberg and Sean Richey, "Anti-Vaccination Beliefs and Unrelated Conspiracy Theories," *World Affairs* 183, no. 2 (2020): 108.

70 Sharon S. Brehm and Jack W. Brehm, *Psychological Reactance: A Theory of Freedom and Control* (New York: Academic Press, 1981), 3–4.

71 Ibid., 4.

72 Hornsey, Harris, and Fielding, "The Psychological Roots of Anti-Vaccination Attitudes: A 24-Nation Investigation."

73 Helps et al., "Understanding Non-Vaccinating Parents' Views to Inform and Improve Clinical Encounters: A Qualitative Study in an Australian Community," 5–6.

74 DoHS, "Government Ends Religious 'No Jab No Pay' of Benefits Exemption," Parliament of Australia, https://parlinfo.aph.gov.au/parlInfo/search/display/display.w3p;query=Id:%22media/pressrel/3783547%22.

75 Sturm, Mays, and Zimet, "Parental Beliefs and Decision Making About Child and Adolescent Immunization: From Polio to Sexually Transmitted Infections."

76 Brewer et al., "Increasing Vaccination: Putting Psychological Science into Action."

77 Browne, "Epistemic Divides and Ontological Confusions: The Psychology of Vaccine Scepticism."; Brunson, "How Parents Make Decisions About Their Children's Vaccinations."

78 Motta et al., "Identifying the Prevalence, Correlates, and Policy Consequences of Anti-Vaccine Social Identity," 2.

79 Brown et al., "UK Parents' Decision-Making About Measles–Mumps–Rubella (MMR) Vaccine 10 Years after the MMR-Autism Controversy: A Qualitative Analysis."; Motta et al., "Identifying the Prevalence, Correlates, and Policy Consequences of Anti-Vaccine Social Identity."

80 Brewer et al., "Increasing Vaccination: Putting Psychological Science into Action," 168.

81 Eve Dubé et al., "Mapping Vaccine Hesitancy—Country-Specific Characteristics of a Global Phenomenon," *Vaccine* 32, no. 49 (2014); Melanie Marti et al., "Assessments of Global Drivers of Vaccine Hesitancy in 2014 – Looking Beyond Safety Concerns," *PLoS One* 12, no. 3 (2017); Michael Favin et al., "Why Children Are Not Vaccinated: A Review of the Grey Literature," *International Health* 4, no. 4 (2012).

82 Tomas Rozbroj, Anthony Lyons, and Jayne Lucke, "Psychosocial and Demographic Characteristics Relating to Vaccine Attitudes in Australia," *Patient Education and Counseling* 102, no. 1 (2019); Thomas Aechtner and Jeremy Farr, "Religion, Trust, and Vaccine Hesitancy in Australia: An Examination of Two Surveys," *Journal for the Academic Study of Religion* 35, no. 2 (2022).

83 N. Fournet et al., "Under-Vaccinated Groups in Europe and Their Beliefs, Attitudes and Reasons for Non-Vaccination; Two Systematic Reviews," *BMC Public Health* 18, no. 1 (2018); Paul G. Van Buynder, "Large Measles Outbreak in a Religious Community in British Columbia," *Journal of Vaccines & Vaccination* 5, no. 5 (2014); C. C. Wielders et al., "Mumps Epidemic in Orthodox Religious Low-Vaccination Communities in the Netherlands and Canada, 2007 to 2009," *Eurosurveillance* 16, no. 41 (2011); Ann Zimmerman and Betsy McKay, "Texas Church Is Center of Measles Outbreak," *The Wall Street Journal*, https://www.wsj.com/articles/texas-church-is-center-of-measles-outbreak-1377646273.

84 John D. Grabenstein, "What the World's Religions Teach, Applied to Vaccines and Immune Globulins," *Vaccine* 31, no. 16 (2013): 2017.

85 Ibid., 2015–16; Charles A. Michael et al., "An Assessment of the Reasons for Oral Poliovirus Vaccine Refusals in Northern Nigeria," *Journal of Infectious Diseases* 210, no. suppl 1 (2014); A. C. de Munter et al., "Decision-Making on Maternal Pertussis Vaccination among Women in a Vaccine-Hesitant Religious Group: Stages and Needs," *PLoS One* 15, no. 11 (2020); Ben Kasstan, "Vaccines and Vitriol: An Anthropological Commentary on Vaccine Hesitancy, Decision-Making and Interventionism among Religious Minorities," *Anthropology & Medicine* 28, no. 4 (2021).

86 Katie E. Corcoran, Christopher P. Scheitle, and Bernard D. DiGregorio, "Christian Nationalism and COVID-19 Vaccine Hesitancy and Uptake," *Vaccine* 39, no. 45 (2021).

87 Sarah J. J. Touyz and Louis Z. G. Touyz, "The Kiss of Death: HPV Rejected by Religion," *Current Oncology* 20, no. 1 (2013); Sharon G. Grossman, "Resolving the Debate over Human Pappiloma Virus (HPV) Vaccination for Cancer Prevention in the Religious World," *Tradition* 51, no. 2 (2019); Julia Bodson et al., "Religion and HPV Vaccine-Related Awareness, Knowledge, and Receipt among Insured Women Aged 18–26 in Utah," *PLoS One* 12, no. 8 (2017).

88 Sabrine Hamdi, "The Impact of Teachings on Sexuality in Islam on HPV Vaccine Acceptability in the Middle East and North Africa Region," *Journal of Epidemiology and Global Health* 7, no. Suppl 1 (2018); Maia Wiesenfeld, "The Infectious Opposition to HPV Vaccination in the Jewish Community," *Derech HaTeva* 21 (2017).

89 Qamar Abbas, Fatima Mangrio, and Sunil Kumar, "Myths, Beliefs, and Conspiracies About COVID-19 Vaccines in Sindh, Pakistan: An Online Crosssectional Survey," *Authorea Preprints* (2021); Kamal-deen O. Sulaiman, "An Assessment of Muslims Reactions to the Immunization of Children in Northern Nigeria," *Medical Journal of Islamic World Academy of Sciences* 22, no. 3 (2014).

90 Ali Ahmed et al., "Outbreak of Vaccine-Preventable Diseases in Muslim Majority Countries," *Journal of Infection and Public Health* 11, no. 2 (2018);

Rubal Kanozia and Ritu Arya, "'Fake News', Religion, and COVID-19 Vaccine Hesitancy in India, Pakistan, and Bangladesh," *Media Asia* 48, no. 4 (2021); Dyna Rochmyaningsih, "Indonesian Fatwa Causes Immunization Rates to Drop," *Science* 362, no. 6415 (2018); Ramadan Mohamed Elkalmi, Shazia Qassim Jamshed, and Azyyati Mohd Suhaimi, "Discrepancies and Similarities in Attitudes, Beliefs, and Familiarity with Vaccination between Religious Studies and Science Students in Malaysia: A Comparison Study," *Journal of Religion and Health* 60, no. 4 (2021).

91   Abbas, Mangrio, and Kumar, "Myths, Beliefs, and Conspiracies About COVID-19 Vaccines in Sindh, Pakistan: An Online Crosssectional Survey."

92   Md Rafiul Biswas et al., "A Scoping Review to Find out Worldwide COVID-19 Vaccine Hesitancy and Its Underlying Determinants," *Vaccines* 9, no. 11 (2021); Fidelia Cascini et al., "Attitudes, Acceptance and Hesitancy among the General Population Worldwide to Receive the COVID-19 Vaccines and Their Contributing Factors: A Systematic Review," *eClinicalMedicine* 40 (2021); Adrian Furnham, "Personal Correlates of Covid-19 Vaccine Hesitancy," *Health* 14 (2022); Mohammad Bellal Hossain et al., "COVID-19 Vaccine Hesitancy among the Adult Population in Bangladesh: A Nationwide Cross-Sectional Survey," *PLoS One* 16, no. 12 (2021); Megan A. Milligan et al., "COVID-19 Vaccine Acceptance: Influential Roles of Political Party and Religiosity," *Psychology, Health & Medicine* (2021); Murphy et al., "Psychological Characteristics Associated with COVID-19 Vaccine Hesitancy and Resistance in Ireland and the United Kingdom."; Ayokunle A. Olagoke, Olakanmi O. Olagoke, and Ashley M. Hughes, "Intention to Vaccinate against the Novel 2019 Coronavirus Disease: The Role of Health Locus of Control and Religiosity," *Journal of Religion and Health* 60, no. 1 (2020); Laura S. Rozek et al., "Understanding Vaccine Hesitancy in the Context of COVID-19: The Role of Trust and Confidence in a Seventeen-Country Survey," *International Journal of Public Health* 66 (2021); Laura Upenieks, Joanne Ford-Robertson, and James E. Robertson, "Trust in God and/or Science? Sociodemographic Differences in the Effects of Beliefs in an Engaged God and Mistrust of the COVID-19 Vaccine," *Journal of Religion and Health* (2021).

93   Timothy Callaghan et al., "Correlates and Disparities of Intention to Vaccinate against COVID-19," *Social Science & Medicine* 272 (2021); David DeFranza et al., "Religion and Reactance to COVID-19 Mitigation Guidelines," *American Psychologist* 76, no. 5 (2021).

94   Aechtner and Farr, "Religion, Trust, and Vaccine Hesitancy in Australia: An Examination of Two Surveys."; Gabriel Andrade, "Vaccine Hesitancy and Religiosity in a Sample of University Students in Venezuela," *Human Vaccines & Immunotherapeutics* (2021); Dan Kahan, "Vaccine Risk Perceptions and Ad Hoc Risk Communication: An Empirical Assessment," in *CCP Risk Perception Studies* (Yale University, 2014); Heidi J. Larson et al., "The State of Vaccine Confidence 2016: Global Insights through a 67-Country Survey," *EBioMedicine* 12, no. C (2016); Joshua T. B. Williams, John D. Rice, and Sean T. O'Leary, "Associations between Religion, Religiosity, and Parental Vaccine Hesitancy," *Vaccine: X* 9 (2021); Aisyah Nur Izzati, Budi Utomo, and Retno Indarwati, "Factors Related to Vaccine Hesitancy in Anti-Vaccine Group on Facebook," *Jurnal Ners* 15, no. 1Sp (2020).

95   Kimmo Eriksson and Irina Vartanova, "Vaccine Confidence Is Higher in More Religious Countries," *Human Vaccines & Immunotherapeutics* Online ahead of print (2021).

96   Paul Bramadat, "Crises of Trust and Truth: Religion, Culture, and Vaccine Hesitancy in Canada," in *Public Health in the Age of Anxiety: Religious and Cultural Roots of Vaccine Hesitancy in Canada*, ed. Paul Bramadat, et al. (Toronto: University of Toronto Press, 2017), 27–28.

97 Eriksson and Vartanova, "Vaccine Confidence Is Higher in More Religious Countries," 1.

98 Gabrielle M. Bryden et al., "Anti-Vaccination and Pro-Cam Attitudes Both Reflect Magical Beliefs About Health," *Vaccine* 36, no. 9 (2018); Aechtner and Farr, "Religion, Trust, and Vaccine Hesitancy in Australia: An Examination of Two Surveys."

99 Stephanie Alice Baker, "Alt. Health Influencers: How Wellness Culture and Web Culture Have Been Weaponised to Promote Conspiracy Theories and Far-Right Extremism During the COVID-19 Pandemic," *European Journal of Cultural Studies* 25, no. 1 (2022); Giovanna Parmigiani, "Magic and Politics: Conspirituality and COVID-19," *Journal of the American Academy of Religion* 89, no. 2 (2021).

100 Esther Chan, "Are the Religious Suspicious of Science? Investigating Religiosity, Religious Context, and Orientations Towards Science," *Public Understanding of Science* 27, no. 8 (2018); Larson et al., "The State of Vaccine Confidence 2016: Global Insights through a 67-Country Survey," 300.

101 Marti et al., "Assessments of Global Drivers of Vaccine Hesitancy in 2014 – Looking Beyond Safety Concerns," 10.

102 Grabenstein, "What the World's Religions Teach, Applied to Vaccines and Immune Globulins"; Richard K. Zimmerman and Jonathan Raviotta, "Steps for Clinicians and Public Health Officials to Take to Reach Persons of Faith, for the Sake of Protecting All against Vaccine-Preventable Diseases," *Vaccine* 31, no. 16.

103 Grabenstein, "What the World's Religions Teach, Applied to Vaccines and Immune Globulins."

104 Ian Glynn and Jenifer Glynn, *The Life and Death of Smallpox* (London: Profile Books, 2004), 112.

105 David P. Mindell, *The Evolving World: Evolution in Everyday Life* (Cambridge: Harvard University Press, 2006), 10.

106 J. L. A. Hautvast et al., "The Role of Religious Leaders in Promoting Acceptance of Vaccination within a Minority Group: A Qualitative Study," *BMC Public Health* 13, no. 1 (2013); J. L. A. Hautvast et al., "How Orthodox Protestant Parents Decide on the Vaccination of Their Children: A Qualitative Study," *BMC Public Health* 12 (2012).

107 Laura A. V. Marlow et al., "Predictors of Interest in HPV Vaccination: A Study of British Adolescents," *Vaccine* 27, no. 18 (2009); Pieter H. Streefland, "Public Doubts About Vaccination Safety and Resistance against Vaccination," *Health Policy* 55, no. 3 (2001).

108 Zimmerman and Raviotta, "Steps for Clinicians and Public Health Officials to Take to Reach Persons of Faith, for the Sake of Protecting All against Vaccine-Preventable Diseases"; Grabenstein, "What the World's Religions Teach, Applied to Vaccines and Immune Globulins."

109 Jason W. Busse, Rishma Walji, and Kumanan Wilson, "Parents' Experiences Discussing Pediatric Vaccination with Healthcare Providers: A Survey of Canadian Naturopathic Patients (Parent Interaction Regarding Pediatric Vaccination)," *PLoS One* 6, no. 8 (2011).

110 Rachel Elizabeth Casiday, "Children's Health and the Social Theory of Risk: Insights from the British Measles, Mumps and Rubella (MMR) Controversy," *Social Science & Medicine* 65, no. 5 (2007); Pru Hobson-West, "Understanding Vaccination Resistance: Moving Beyond Risk," *Health, Risk & Society* 5, no. 3 (2003).

111 Streefland, Chowdhury, and Ramos-Jimenez, "Patterns of Vaccination Acceptance."

112 María D. Esteban-Vasallo et al., "Adequacy of Information Provided by Healthcare Professionals on Vaccines: Results of a Population Survey in

Spain," *Patient Education and Counseling* 101, no. 7 (2018); Brown et al., "UK Parents' Decision-Making About Measles–Mumps–Rubella (MMR) Vaccine 10 Years after the MMR-Autism Controversy: A Qualitative Analysis."

113 J. Leask et al., "Communicating with Parents About Vaccination: A Framework for Health Professionals," *BMC Pediatrics* 12, no. 1 (2012).

114 Narayan and Preljevic, "An Information Behaviour Approach to Conspiracy Theories: Listening in on Voices from within the Vaccination Debate."; Betsch and Sachse, "Dr. Jekyll or Mr. Hyde."; Kata, "A Postmodern Pandora's Box: Anti-Vaccination Misinformation on the Internet."

115 Aechtner, "Improving Evolution Advocacy: Translating Vaccine Interventions to the Evolution Wars."

116 Kata, "A Postmodern Pandora's Box: Anti-Vaccination Misinformation on the Internet."; Wolfe, "Vaccine Safety Activists on the Internet."; Richard Zimmerman et al., "Vaccine Criticism on the World Wide Web," *Journal of Medical Internet Research* 7, no. 2 (2005).

117 Vernon, "Is Vaccine Dissent Based on Science?"; Heller, "Trust in Institutions, Science"; Anna Kata, "Anti-Vaccine Activists, Web 2.0, and the Postmodern Paradigm – an Overview of Tactics and Tropes Used Online by the Anti-Vaccination Movement," *Vaccine* 30, no. 25 (2012); Davies, Chapman, and Leask, "Antivaccination Activists on the World Wide Web."

118 Kahan et al., "Geoengineering and Climate Change Polarization."

119 Dan Kahan, "Cultural Cognition as a Conception of the Cultural Theory of Risk," in *Handbook of Risk Theory: Epistemology, Decision Theory, Ethics, and Social Implications of Risk*, ed. Sabine Roeser, et al. (Dordrecht: Springer, 2012), 740.

120 Ibid.

121 Dan Kahan and Donald Braman, "The Self-Defensive Cognition of Self-Defense," *The American Criminal Law Review* 45, no. 1 (2008): 5.

122 Dan Kahan et al., "Who Fears the HPV Vaccine, Who Doesn't, and Why?: An Experimental Study of the Mechanisms of Cultural Cognition," *Law and Human Behavior* 34, no. 6 (2010): 502.

123 Kahan, "Cultural Cognition," 740.

124 Dan M. Kahan, Hank Jenkins-Smith, and Donald Braman, "Cultural Cognition of Scientific Consensus," *Journal of Risk Research* 14, no. 2 (2011): 149–50.

125 Dan Kahan, "Making Climate-Science Communication Evidence-Based: All the Way Down," in *Culture, Politics and Climate Change: How Information Shapes Our Common Future*, ed. Deserai A. Crow and Maxwell T. Boykoff (Abingdon: Routledge, 2014), 209.

126 Adapted from Kahan, "Cultural Cognition," 732.

127 Ibid., 731.

128 Ibid.

129 Ibid.

130 Ibid.

131 Kahan, "Making Climate-Science Communication."

132 Ibid.

133 Alessandro Germani et al., "Emerging Adults and COVID-19: The Role of Individualism-Collectivism on Perceived Risks and Psychological Maladjustment," *International Journal of Environmental Research and Public Health* 17, no. 10 (2020); Jeroen Luyten et al., "Kicking against the Pricks: Vaccine Sceptics Have a Different Social Orientation," *European Journal of Public Health* 24, no. 2 (2014); Laura J. Holt, Dina Anselmi, and Skye A. Gasataya, "Predictors of Vaccine Hesitancy in College-Attending Emerging Adults: Implications for Public Health Outreach," *American Journal of Health Education* 53, no. 3 (2022).

134 Harry Charalambos Triandis, *Individualism & Collectivism* (Boulder: Westview Press, 1995), 43.

135 Luyten et al., "Kicking against the Pricks: Vaccine Sceptics Have a Different Social Orientation"; Holt, Anselmi, and Gasataya, "Predictors of Vaccine Hesitancy in College-Attending Emerging Adults: Implications for Public Health Outreach."

136 Triandis, *Individualism & Collectivism*, 43.

137 Luyten et al., "Kicking against the Pricks: Vaccine Sceptics Have a Different Social Orientation"; Holt, Anselmi, and Gasataya, "Predictors of Vaccine Hesitancy in College-Attending Emerging Adults: Implications for Public Health Outreach."

138 Kahan, "Cultural Cognition," 752.

139 Marc Hauser et al., "A Dissociation between Moral Judgments and Justifications," *Mind & Language* 22, no. 1 (2007): 17–18.

140 Jonathan Haidt and Jesse Graham, "When Morality Opposes Justice: Conservatives Have Moral Intuitions That Liberals May Not Recognize," *Social Justice Research* 20, no. 1 (2007): 104–06; Jonathan Haidt, *The Righteous Mind: Why Good People Are Divided by Politics and Religion*, 1st edn. (New York: Pantheon Books, 2012).

141 Ibid.

142 Ibid.

143 Ibid.

144 Ibid.

145 Ibid.

146 Ibid.; Ravi Iyer et al., "Understanding Libertarian Morality: The Psychological Dispositions of Self-Identified Libertarians," *PLoS One* 7, no. 8 (2012).

147 Jesse Graham et al., "Moral Foundations Theory: The Pragmatic Validity of Moral Pluralism," in *Advances in Experimental Social Psychology*, ed. Patricia Devine and Ashby Plant (Oxford: Elsevier Science, 2013), 63–65.

148 Christopher Suhler and Patricia Churchland, "Can Innate, Modular 'Foundations' Explain Morality? Challenges for Haidt's Moral Foundations Theory," *Journal of Cognitive Neuroscience* 23, no. 9 (2011).

149 L. Dickinson Janis et al., "Which Moral Foundations Predict Willingness to Make Lifestyle Changes to Avert Climate Change in the USA?," *PLoS One* 11, no. 10 (2016); Avnika B. Amin et al., "Association of Moral Values with Vaccine Hesitancy," *Nature Human Behaviour* 1, no. 12 (2017); Matthew Feinberg and Robb Willer, "From Gulf to Bridge: When Do Moral Arguments Facilitate Political Influence?," *Personality and Social Psychology Bulletin* 41, no. 12 (2015).

150 Jesse Graham, Jonathan Haidt, and Brian A. Nosek, "Liberals and Conservatives Rely on Different Sets of Moral Foundations," *Journal of Personality and Social Psychology* 96, no. 5 (2009): 1040.

151 Janis et al., "Which Moral Foundations Predict," 3; Haidt and Graham, "When Morality Opposes Justice."

152 Christopher Wolsko, Hector Ariceaga, and Jesse Seiden, "Red, White, and Blue Enough to Be Green: Effects of Moral Framing on Climate Change Attitudes and Conservation Behaviors," *Journal of Experimental Social Psychology* 65 (2016).

153 Amin et al., "Association of Moral Values," 876.

154 Ibid., 877.

155 Isabel Rossen et al., "Accepters, Fence Sitters, or Rejecters: Moral Profiles of Vaccination Attitudes," *Social Science & Medicine* 224 (2019).

156 John Philip Jones, ed. *How Advertising Works: The Role of Research* (Thousand Oaks: Sage Publications, 1998).

157   Edwin Emery, "Changing Role of the Mass Media in American Politics," *Annals of the American Academy of Political and Social Science* 427 (1976); Michael M. Franz and Travis N. Ridout, "Does Political Advertising Persuade?," *Political Behavior* 29, no. 4 (2007); Gregory A. Huber and Kevin Arceneaux, "Identifying the Persuasive Effects of Presidential Advertising," *American Journal of Political Science* 51, no. 4 (2007); Jenny Lloyd, "Positively Negative: The Impact of Negativity Upon the Political Consumer," *International Journal of Nonprofit and Voluntary Sector Marketing* 13 (2008); Agnieszka Dobrzynska, André Blais, and Richard Nadeau, "Do the Media Have a Direct Impact on the Vote?: The Case of the 1997 Canadian Election," *International Journal of Public Opinion Research* 15, no. 1 (2003); Julie M. Duck, Michael A. Hogg, and Deborah J. Terry, "Me, Us and Them: Political Identification and the Third-Person Effect in the 1993 Australian Federal Election," *European Journal of Social Psychology* 25, no. 2 (1995); Brandon S. Centerwall, "Television and Violence: The Scale of the Problem and Where to Go from Here," *The Journal of the American Medical Association* 267, no. 22 (1992); Richard B. Felson, "Mass Media Effects on Violent Behavior," *Annual Review of Sociology* 22 (1996); Linda Heath, Linda B. Bresolin, and Robert C. Rinaldi, "Effects of Media Violence on Children: A Review of the Literature," *Archives of General Psychiatry* 46, no. 4 (1989); L. Rowell Huesmann et al., "Longitudinal Relations between Children's Exposure to TV Violence and Their Aggressive and Violent Behavior in Young Adulthood: 1977–1992," *Developmental Psychology* 39, no. 2 (2003); L. Rowell Huesmann and Laramie D. Taylor, "The Role of Media Violence in Violent Behavior," *Annual Review of Public Health* 27 (2006); Haejung Paik and George Comstock, "The Effects of Television Violence on Antisocial Behavior: A Meta-Analysis," *Communication Research* 21, no. 4 (1994); David K. Perry, *Theory and Research in Mass Communication: Contexts and Consequences*, 2nd ed. (Mahwah: Lawrence Erlbaum Associates, 2002); Glenn G. Sparks and Cheri W. Sparks, "Effects of Media Violence," in *Media Effects: Advances in Theory and Research*, ed. Jennings Bryant and Dolf Zillmann (Mahwah: Lawrence Erlbaum, 2002); Wendy Wood, Frank Y. Wonga, and J.Gregory Chacherea, "Effects of Media Violence on Viewers' Aggression in Unconstrained Social Interaction," *Psychological Bulletin* 109, no. 3 (1991); Akinrinola Bankole, German Rodriguez, and Charles Westoff, "Mass Media Messages and Reproductive Behavior in Nigeria," *Journal of Biosocial Science* 28, no. 2 (1996); Jennifer S. Barber and William G. Axinn, "New Ideas and Fertility Limitation: The Role of Mass Media," *Journal of Marriage and Family* 66, no. 5 (2004); Neeru Gupta, Charles Katende, and Ruth Bessinger, "Associations of Mass Media Exposure with Family Planning Attitudes and Practices in Uganda," *Studies in Family Planning* 34, no. 1 (2003); Robert C. Hornik, ed. *Public Health Communication: Evidence for Behavior Change* (Mahwah: Lawrence Erlbaum, 2002); Roger H. Secker-Walker et al., "A Mass Media Programme to Prevent Smoking among Adolescents: Costs and Cost Effectiveness," *Tobacco Control* 6, no. 3 (1997).

158   Robert Levine, *The Power of Persuasion: How We're Bought and Sold* (New Jersey: John Wiley & Sons, 2003), 18; Franz and Ridout, "Does Political," 465–66; Jason Motlagh, "Why the Taliban Is Winning the Propaganda War," *Time*, https://content.time.com/time/world/article/0,8599,1895496,00.html.

159   W. Davison, "The Third-Person Effect in Communication," *Public Opinion Quarterly* 47, no. 1 (1983).

160   Timothy W. McGuire, "Measuring and Testing Relative Advertising Effectiveness with Split-Cable TV Panel Data," *Journal of the American Statistical Association* 72, no. 360 (1977); Magid M. Abraham and Leonard M. Lodish, "Getting the Most out of Advertising and Promotion," *Harvard Business*

Review 68, no. 3 (1990); Leonard M. Lodish et al., "How T.V. Advertising Works: A Meta-Analysis of 389 Real World Split Cable T.V. Advertising Experiments," *Journal of Marketing Research* 32, no. 2 (1995); William D. Wells, ed. *Measuring Advertising Effectiveness* (Mahwah: Lawrence Erlbaum, 1997); Levine, *The Power of Persuasion*, 24–28; Karen E. Dill, *How Fantasy Becomes Reality: Seeing through Media Influence* (New York: Oxford University Press, 2009).

161 Adapted from Richard E. Petty and John T. Cacioppo, *Communication and Persuasion: Central and Peripheral Routes to Attitude Change* (New York: Springer-Verlag, 1986), 4.

162 "The Effects of Involvement on Responses to Argument Quantity and Quality: Central and Peripheral Routes to Persuasion," *Journal of Personality and Social Psychology* 46, no. 1 (1984): 70.

163 Ibid.

164 Petty and Cacioppo, *Communication and Persuasion*, 142.

165 Phyllis A. Anastasio, Karen C. Rose, and Judith Chapman, "Can the Media Create Public Opinion? A Social-Identity Approach," *Current Directions in Psychological Science* 8, no. 5 (1999): 154.

166 Petty and Cacioppo, *Communication and Persuasion*, 18.

167 Ibid., 23; Anastasio, Rose, and Chapman, "Can the Media Create Public Opinion?," 154; Elizabeth M. Perse, *Media Effects and Society* (Mahwah: Lawrence Erlbaum Associates, 2001), 85–86; Richard E. Petty, Joseph R. Priester, and Pablo Brinol, "Mass Media Attitude Change: Implications of the Elaboration Likelihood Model of Persuasion," in *Media Effects: Advances in Theory and Research*, ed. Jennings Bryant and Dolf Zillmann (Mahwah: Lawrence Erlbaum, 2002), 168.

168 Petty and Cacioppo, *Communication and Persuasion*, 24; Richard E. Petty, Curtis P. Haugtvedt, and Stephen M. Smith, "Elaboration as a Determinant of Attitude Strength: Creating Attitudes That Are Persistent, Resistant, and Predictive of Behavior," in *Attitude Strength: Antecedents and Consequences*, ed. Richard E. Petty and Jon A. Krosnick (Mahwah: Lawrence Erlbaum, 1995), 93–130.

169 Paul W. Miniard, Deepak Sirdeshmukh, and Daniel E. Innis, "Peripheral Persuasion and Brand Choice," *Journal of Consumer Research* 19, no. 2 (1992); Paul W. Miniard et al., "Picture-Based Persuasion Processes and the Moderating Role of Involvement," *Journal of Consumer Research* 18, no. 1 (1991); Richard E. Petty, John T. Cacioppo, and David Schumann, "Central and Peripheral Routes to Advertising Effectiveness: The Moderating Role of Involvement," *Journal of Consumer Research* 10, no. 2 (1983).

3   Suspicious hesitancy
Distrust and Confidence

Vaccine hesitancy is more complicated than it might appear at first glance. Vaccination decision-making has also proven to be surprisingly knotty and involves several variables beyond simply people's knowledge about vaccines. On top of these realities is the fact that committed vaccine deniers and vaccine hesitant individuals come from a variety of sociocultural circumstances, and they do not belong to a single uniform group. They can represent thoroughly different demographics, with dissimilar socioeconomic backgrounds, beliefs, education levels, and life experiences. Yet, amongst all these complexities is a single, clear overarching fact. This is that anti-vaccination arguments and persuasion strategies are often remarkably similar. Many of the same counter-immunisation notions, and repeated challenges to vaccines can be identified around the world, throughout history. These contentions tend to revolve around a nucleus of common themes, which can be labelled as the *Distrust, Confidence*, and *Danger* motifs. This chapter will introduce each of these themes, and then break down in greater detail specifically the Distrust and Confidence categories. With respect to these categories, the chapter will also introduce five vaccination myths associated with the Distrust and Confidence themes, as well four persuasive cues that frequently appear in antivaccination arguments.

Introducing the DCD of antivaccination messages

Antivaccine messages are typically established upon Distrust, Confidence, and Danger claims. These can be abbreviated as the *DCD* of antivaccination communications. The first theme in this abbreviation is particularly important, because feelings of distrust have been repeatedly found to be associated with vaccine misgivings and immunisation rejection. The Distrust motif in counter-vaccine assertions taps into these feelings, as it largely involves claims about pro-vaccine conspiracies. Such accounts detail apparent coverups of vaccine dangers for the sake of profit, as well as allegations of suppression efforts to muffle counter-vaccine evidence. This theme incorporates claims that governments are restricting our personal freedoms by mandating population-wide vaccination efforts. It also features attempts to cast doubt upon experts, as well as attempts to

DOI: 10.4324/9781003312550-3

spread misgivings about the science and safety of vaccines. In this way, the Distrust theme often involves questioning established consensus science, and challenging the motivations of corporations and scientists, the legitimacy of governments, and the authority of healthcare professionals. The target of Distrust messages includes everyone who may be involved in producing, testing, monitoring, and administering vaccines, as well as officials setting vaccine public policy.

The next theme, described as Confidence, underlines the personal expertise of people who are sceptical of vaccines, and the credentials of apparent specialists opposed to vaccinating. This theme can involve accentuating the science that is claimed to back up antivaccination arguments, while also focussing on the number of other people who are said to support counter-vaccine initiatives. In a sense, the Confidence theme counterbalances Distrust claims. While Distrust messages dispute experts and facts, the Confidence theme involves attempts to tell people who they should really trust instead of the scientific consensus and leading authorities. The Confidence element of antivaccine messages affirms that members of the public should trust their own expertise, their own experiences, and their own research. It asserts that people should base their opinions on the alleged science and scientific experts who are said to dispute the safety and effectiveness of vaccines.

Finally, the Danger theme of the DCD acronym is concentrated upon vaccination fears. It includes publicising alleged vaccination risks that can involve a variety of frightening side effects, along with stories about vaccines causing autism or even death. These fear-linked reports are often communicated through firsthand personal narratives, which can involve references to the effects of seemingly toxic, untested vaccine ingredients. Such anxiety garnering narratives are widespread, on and offline, and no matter what our opinion of vaccines might be, it is likely we have heard tales of vaccine-related injury from friends and family. Many of these claims are fabricated and scientifically unsubstantiated. However, it is critical to remember that such arguments can be influential, and that antivaccination media is often laden with persuasive messaging in ways that pro-vaccine communications are not.[1]

Notably, Distrust, Confidence, and Danger claims can together capitalise upon the central reasons influencing the likelihood of getting vaccinated described in the previous chapter. For instance, the Danger theme addresses people's vaccine fears and risk calculations. Distrust plotlines, on the other hand, may resonate with individuals who are questioning vaccine effectiveness. They could also appeal to people who are already sceptical about pharmaceutical companies and consensus science, and those more open to conspiratorial ideas about authorities and corporations. The Distrust theme may further connect with people whose beliefs and values are opposed to mandatory vaccination laws. At the same time, the Confidence motif can assure people that they can trust their own expertise and life history, where personal experiences may deeply shape vaccination decision-making. Furthermore, the DCD are embedded in counter-vaccine media, and such media is often an ingredient in fostering vaccine doubts. Altogether then, the Distrust, Confidence, and Danger themes are more than simple rhetoric. This is because they also can reflect key justifications and motivations that have been found to underpin people's choices to not get vaccinated.

Focusing on distrust

Feelings of distrust have consistently been associated with vaccine hesitancy and lower vaccine uptake. This distrust can stem from a shortage of confidence in government, healthcare workers, and vaccine manufacturers.[2] Antivaccination social media is also brimming with distrustful posts, and ardent vaccine refusers tend to voice substantial suspicions.[3] As a study concluded, "One thing we do know is that doctors (in general) and pharmaceutical companies (en masse) are distrusted by vaccine rejecting parents."[4] Additionally, for some, such distrust can be influenced by, and spill into, conspiratorial ways of thinking and the acceptance of conspiracy theories.[5] Conspiracy theories can be described as attempts to explain events as the result of schemes carried out by powerful individuals, who are concealing their role behind malevolent agendas.[6] By no means does this suggest that vaccine hesitancy is synonymous with accepting conspiracy theories. However, it is evident that many antivaccine messages tap into prevalent feelings of distrust and inclinations toward conspiracist ideas by actively distributing conspiracy narratives.[7]

The central method by which antivaccination media often plays upon public distrust is by claiming that governments are tyrannically trying to restrict people's medical autonomy and citizen's personal health choices by making vaccination mandatory.[8] Additionally, counter-vaccine messages repeatedly claim that scientific data about vaccine risks, and the true harm that vaccines cause, are actively being suppressed by governments and pharmaceutical companies in a conspiracy to make money. This international conspiracy involves covering up stories from across the globe about people being injured or even killed by vaccines.[9] Accordingly, a fundamental characteristic of antivaccination communications is that they are often concentrated upon provoking distrust of medical and governmental authorities, and these distrust messages are frequently expressed through conspiratorial storylines.

What is significant is that conspiracy theories seem to be stubbornly persuasive. This observation has driven researchers to uncover why they can be so convincing to so many people. Various studies have pointed to the fact that conspiracy theories seem to fill a psychological need when people feel powerless, voiceless, as well as when they believe that there is not enough clear, understandable information to explain events.[10] Conspiratorial beliefs tend to increase when people experience "fear, uncertainty, and the feeling of being out of control" as a result of societal crises.[11] These feelings can prompt individuals to accept conspiracy theories to make sense of such predicaments. As Victoria Pagán has noted, conspiracy theories meet the "challenge of the lack of knowledge with a preponderance of explanation."[12] These trends can apply to personal crises as well, including the diagnosis of autism in one's child. Such incidents can be difficult to make sense of, and conspiracy theories may soothe feelings of helplessness. They might offer a rekindled level of perceived understanding, and a sense of control when seemingly incomprehensible situations occur.[13] It is also thought that conspiratorial narratives aid in protecting people's self-esteem when they try to make sense of their failures in meeting goals.[14] If someone has failed in achieving an objective, or a movement has been unsuccessful in obtaining its goals, a conspiracy can deflect blame for the disappointment, and protect self-image by holding someone else responsible.[15]

Taken as a whole, conspiracy theories serve as psychological coping mechanisms in times of fear, disappointment, stress, and uncertainty.[16] Conspiracies have also been linked to more intuitive styles of thinking rather than analytical modes of thought.[17] Intuitive thinking relies more on emotions and quick decision-making using gut feelings. Links have further been identified between lower levels of interpersonal trust and belief in conspiracies.[18] It is also thought that conspiracy theories can satisfy people's "need for uniqueness," because they can make some individuals feel part of an enlightened group that has privileged access to extraordinary information. By having an inside track to the conspiracy story, people can gain a sense of holding special insider knowledge that the rest of the population is blind to or not willing to accept.[19]

Ultimately, conspiracy theories harness people's distrust of official sources of knowledge, including governments, medical workers, and academics. When it comes to antivaccination media, audiences are told to actively question the experts, and not to simply trust advice from authorities. People are also encouraged to resist being told what to do by experts and governments when it comes to vaccination choices. Antivaccination media, therefore, often alleges conspiracies, while it can further assert that mandatory vaccination programs are coercive and infringe upon our civil liberties. People are instructed that such policies are being enacted by untrustworthy people in high places who are limiting our freedoms for conspiratorial gain.[20] Such messages of coercion and the perception that vaccination choices are forcibly being limited, perhaps via a grand conspiratorial plot, can also induce psychological reactance (Chapter 2). These considerations should not be overlooked, because scholars have pointed out that many people today are no longer willing to just accept directives from experts and authorities in power. As one researcher has stated:

> The times when we were simply, even blindly, expected to trust people *because* they were in positions of power has gone. This is not to

say that people in power should not be trusted, but simply that people are expected to question such authority, access other sources of information and perform the role of the "informed citizen". Across many countries and cultures, this unquestioning of power has been somewhat eroded and, in some cases, broken. This is certainly the case for some, although a minority, of parents who actively distrust childhood vaccinations.[21]

It is for all these reasons that antivaccination messages featuring conspiracy messages with warnings to be distrustful of the experts, and claims that governments are taking away health choices, can be surprisingly persuasive.[22] In relation to this persuasiveness, there are several vaccine myths and key persuasive cues that relate to the Distrust theme in antivaccination arguments. A predominant, but catchy conspiratorial fiction, is that vaccines are substantially lucrative for developers and medical providers.

Myth #1: Vaccines are major money-makers for BigPharma, government, and doctors

It has been claimed that "Conspiratorial thinking is endemic in anti-vaccination groups."[23] At the heart of the conspiratorial ideas that are expressed throughout antivaccination media are tales about untrustworthy pharmaceutical companies, governments, and healthcare practitioners profiting financially from vaccines. Allegedly, the pursuit of such profit has led Big-Pharma and authorities to cover up the harm that vaccines cause and hide the fact that vaccines may not be particularly effective. It has also led governments to forcefully push vaccines onto citizens by enforcing mandatory vaccination policies. What are we to make of these assertions?

From the outset, it must be acknowledged that pharmaceutical companies *do* make money from the sale of vaccines. Some people might be uneasy with that reality, but profit-making does not automatically imply that something crooked is necessarily occurring, or that there is a far-reaching conspiracy to cover up the risks and uselessness of vaccines. Companies profit from making abundant types of medicines and medical equipment all around the globe. Such income does not signify that medicines and medical equipment are dangerous, ineffective, or that there are conspiracies occurring to ensure that such products are being sold. For example, surgeons wear face masks during operations to protect patients from pathogens that might be present in the surgical staff's saliva, facial hair, or nasal passages. Such masks also reciprocally protect healthcare workers from a patient's bodily fluids. There are companies that profit from making surgical face masks explicitly for these purposes. However, profit-making does not inevitably denote that the masks are ineffective or dangerous. Making a profit also does not suggest that there is a conspiracy orchestrated by mask manufacturers to ensure that people are getting sick and requiring surgeries so that the companies can keep making financial returns. Likewise, it does not necessarily follow that pharmaceutical companies making money from vaccines is indicative of dishonest activities. Instead, it points to the fact that if pharmaceutical companies *did not* make some money from the production of vaccines, they would likely not remain in the business.

The question then arises regarding how much money pharmaceutical companies earn from producing vaccines. Vaccines have a profit margin of approximately 3%, which is relatively low in comparison to pharmaceuticals used to treat disease.[24] Vaccines are simply not the most commercial products developed by pharmaceutical companies. This is because they can be laborious to manufacture, resulting in higher production costs. They are also heavily regulated and often result in low sale prices. In fact, it has been estimated that vaccines represent only 2–3% of the global pharmaceutical market.[25] As a result, vaccines are a far less attractive business venture than producing other medicines, since vaccines require expensive and complex means of production with the prospect of lower profit margins, strict regulations, while they are also used to prevent disease rather than treating diseases after infection.

What about the likelihood of medical practitioners and government profiting from vaccinating the public? Research has found that the expenses related to administering vaccines, which include supply costs, expenditures of time spent with patients, as well as medical disposal charges total more than what healthcare practitioners are reimbursed for providing vaccinations.[26] As a matter of fact, the ratio of reimbursement-to-costs of giving vaccines has been identified as a potential hindrance that may disincentivise healthcare professionals from offering vaccines to patients.[27] As one study concluded, many doctors receive "little or no profit from vaccine delivery," and instead "most practices lose money" in order to administer vaccines.[28]

Governments, on the other hand, are responsible for supplying vaccines to their populations. Their goal is to reduce prices so that they can secure the most vaccine doses for the greatest number of individuals. Governments are also spending appreciable sums regulating and monitoring vaccine safety (Chapter 1). Many political authorities further provide some financial incentives for doctors to administer vaccines, and to follow-up with overdue patients who may be behind on their vaccinations.[29] This can help ease the financial burden that doctors face in relation to vaccination costs. Consequently, doctors are not profiting from administering vaccines. Moreover, governments are expending funds rather than benefiting financially, to secure population health through vaccination, including dispensing healthcare incentives needed by medical practitioners to fund their vaccination efforts.

For these reasons, an important question to consider is why would pharmaceutical companies engage in a wide-reaching, theoretically expensive, and time-consuming international conspiracy to protect what amounts to only 2–3% of the worldwide pharmaceutical sector? Also, if vaccines result in roughly 3% profit margins for the pharmaceutical sector, there is not a vast money-making surplus for doctors and governments to cash in on, even if they were colluding with BigPharma. Furthermore, as researchers have shown, doctors are often losing capital by administering vaccines. There is little monetary incentive for medical practitioners to vaccinate patients, aside from ensuring the health of the communities that they serve. The myth that vaccines are major money-makers for BigPharma, government, and doctors proves to be shaky ground upon which many antivaccination conspiracy narratives are built.

Distrust and the Scarcity Principle

An underlying characteristic of the antivaccination Distrust theme involves repeated allegations that vaccine truths are being hidden, and that our freedoms are being taken away from us. This can include assertions that scientific data about the real dangers of vaccines are being withheld, that antivaccinationists are being censored by corrupt forces, and that our civil liberties are being undemocratically restricted by mandatory vaccination policies. As one antivaccination leader has stated, "Today, more then [*sic*] ever, the government and the medical community are trying to restrict your right to make informed health choices for yourself and your family."[30]

These claims tend to be linked to conspiratorial plotlines that underpin many antivaccination messages. They also match up with the persuasive cue known as the *Scarcity Principle*. This cue is based upon the simple fact that "we can often use an item's availability to help us quickly and correctly decide on its quality."[31] In relation to the Elaboration Likelihood Model of persuasion, research has demonstrated that when an item appears to be in limited supply its scarcity can act as a compelling peripheral shortcut, causing its perceived value and appeal to be greatly increased.[32] As Jae Min Jung and James J. Kellaris explain, "Because valuable objects are often scarce, people tend to infer that scarce objects are valuable," and subsequently, consumers "often infer value in a product that has limited availability or is promoted as being scarce."[33] Similarly, when items or ideas are banned or censored, people's appetites for these items and ideas can become intensified due to their perceived scarcity.[34] Even the suggestion that information is being suppressed by a certain party can increase an audience's thirst for the data apparently being suppressed. This significantly increases persuasion towards the censored information, even if audience members initially disagreed with the suppressed position.

The power of scarcity claims involving censorship can be located in their ability to induce psychological reactance, which provokes individuals to re-establish threatened liberties.[35] One such reactance response includes the increased attractiveness of a censored product, information, or actions.[36] Accordingly, if audiences are informed that certain facts or choices are being restricted, the appeal of the censored information, as well as the desire to restore access to it, can become amplified. People also seem more likely to react negatively to instructions when they are given as forceful commands, because strict orders are sometimes interpreted as a threat to people's freedom.[37] With all this in mind, one antivaccinationist media maker has stated, the "harder doctors and government officials try to push and the more they try to suppress information and force complaince [*sic*], the more they will find that people are saying no – even if saying no means losing their job."[38] For these reasons, it is important to look out for assertions that facts are being concealed, that the truth is being muzzled, and that your rights are being abolished. These are examples of the Scarcity Principle and its persuasive influences at work in counter-vaccine messages.[39]

Empowering audiences through Distrust

Alongside cases of the Scarcity Principle, antivaccination messages repetitively plead with audiences to defend the truth, and to seek out the "genuine facts" about vaccines for themselves. Counter-vaccine communicators often caution people to avoid being dictated to by untrustworthy authorities, who are censoring data and taking away their rights. In this way, antivaccination media can be infused with an additional level of persuasion, because it empowers and emboldens people to question official sources of knowledge; to seek out the truth, to hear all sides of the story, and to think with an open mind about the data. As Masaryk and Hatoková have explained:

> When we contrast the way in which pro-vaccination and anti-vaccination messages are communicated, the latter seem to empower their audience by asking them to avoid being manipulated, by focusing on positive values such as freedom, or by helping them uncover links between medicine and the pharmaceutical business. This places the individual in a position of strength: by doing something as relatively simple as rejecting vaccination, they can actually grow stronger in their position of relative vulnerability against the powerful and sometimes confusing position of the state in vaccination policy.[40]

Antivaccination media does not simply claim that there is a conspiratorial cover-up. It also empowers audiences to fight for civic freedoms, to make up their own minds, and to unearth the truth for themselves with their own research. Unfortunately, such research is often conducted online, which can expose people to vaccine myths, including the belief that vaccination is unnecessary when infection rates are low.

Myth #2: Low infections make vaccines unnecessary

In many countries society-wide vaccination has helped to reduce infection rates, or even eliminate endemic cases of vaccine-preventable diseases. As a result, some people assume that because such diseases appear so rarely in their communities, vaccines are no longer necessary. Unfortunately, there are several difficulties with such an assumption, and the case of the measles virus demonstrates the myth's problems. In 2000, measles was officially declared to have been eliminated from the USA. This meant that the nation had eradicated endemic measles across the country.[41] Other nations have been able to achieve similar results with widespread vaccination campaigns. Canada eliminated measles in 1998, while in 2014 the World Health Organization declared Australia to be free of endemic measles.[42] However, in the years following each of these declarations, outbreaks of the highly infectious virus occurred within all three countries, as well as in other nations around the globe that had previously stamped out measles within their borders. These outbreaks resulted from unvaccinated travellers, who were infected overseas and returned with the highly communicable illness. When these individuals arrived back to communities exhibiting relatively low measles vaccination rates, the virus was then able to spread.

The story of outbreaks following the eradication of measles exhibits why low infection rates do not make vaccines unnecessary, even for diseases that some people have never experienced before. The reason why measles was eradicated from many countries in the first place was because of the effectiveness of measles vaccines. Many people simply do not witness cases of measles-linked morbidity and mortality for themselves due to such vaccination efforts.[43] However, when people stop receiving the measles vaccine and the disease is reintroduced by travellers, the virus will again spread and cause sickness. In fact, a small number of measles cases could swiftly multiply to thousands of infections if enough individuals in a given population are not vaccinated. High vaccination rates from diseases we do not regularly encounter keeps this from happening, while vaccines also protect immunocompromised individuals and those who are unable to get vaccinated.

This myth is complicated by the fact that vaccine preventable diseases like measles are still active throughout the world today. For instance, the World Health Organization reported that more than 140,000 people died from measles in 2018.[44] Most of these deaths occurred in children under five years of age. Also, "Babies and very young children are at greatest risk from measles infections, with potential complications including pneumonia and encephalitis (a swelling of the brain), as well as lifelong disability – permanent brain damage, blindness or hearing loss."[45] Vaccine preventable diseases pose an ongoing risk, even in countries where the pathogen has been endemically eradicated. This is because such avoidable illnesses still exist elsewhere, meaning that there is an ongoing risk that can be reintroduced.

This stark reality was made clear after several countries went on to lose their measles elimination status.[46] These nations lost this coveted standing when resurgences of measles caused lingering outbreaks involving sustained transmission for more than a year. Such countries have included Brazil, Greece, and the United Kingdom, while in 2019 the USA "narrowly missed losing its elimination status, following its largest measles outbreak since it achieved elimination in 2000."[47] These cases reinforce that "while measles elimination is hard won, it can be easily lost," and they should serve as a "wake-up call," to remind us that even when local infections are low, the need for vaccines remains high.[48] They also constitute evidence about problems associated with the next vaccine myth: that it was not vaccines that controlled vaccine-preventable diseases, but good hygiene, sanitation, clean water, and nutrition.

Myth #3: Better hygiene, sanitation, and nutrition not vaccines

While some people believe that getting vaccinated today is unnecessary because local infection rates are low, it has also been stated that improved hygiene, sanitation, and nutrition, along with the development of antibiotics, were truly responsible for reducing infectious diseases. This argument suggests that a combination of these factors, rather than vaccines themselves, explain declines in illnesses throughout history. It has been argued that vaccination "could not have played a major role in health as often claimed."[49] What is notable about such contentions is that there is an element of truth woven into this myth. Better hygiene, sanitation, nutrition and the use of antibiotics *do* improve community health. Nevertheless, they also do not fully account for declines in infectious diseases that have resulted from vaccines.

Without doubt, better hygiene, sanitation, nutrition, and access to antibiotics all play important roles in improving public health. For instance, access to clean water, hygienic practices, and sanitation facilities can prevent serious illnesses, including diarrheal diseases caused by cholera, dysentery, and typhoid. As Kenneth A. Reinert has explained, diarrheal diseases "are one of the leading causes of infant and child deaths in the world, estimated to account for approximately 9 percent of total infant and child mortality or 580,000 infants and children a year."[50] In fact, the United Nations has reported that every single day "nearly 1,000 children die due to preventable water and sanitation-related diarrheal diseases."[51] It is with this in mind that Reinert has asserted, "A rule of thumb is that improved sanitation could reduce child diarrheal deaths by one third."[52] When we add the influences of nutrition and antibiotics, it is clear that such factors can have definitive health benefits. It is also the case that certain diseases had already been in decline across parts of the world prior to the introduction of vaccinations because of sanitation, hygiene, and nutrition enhancements.

Nevertheless, these truths do not lessen the genuine impact that vaccines have had in preventing disease. Though hygiene, sanitation, nutrition, and the availability of antibiotics can radically impact health, reductions in mortality from such illnesses as diphtheria, measles, polio, smallpox and tetanus greatly decreased following vaccination efforts. Furthermore, it is evident that the introduction of vaccines in nations which possessed first-rate living conditions still led to rapid declines in infections. These positive outcomes resulted from vaccines, because sanitation and good hygiene standards had long since been well established. An example of this includes the Haemophilus Influenzae Type B (Hib) vaccine introduced in 1993. At the time that the Hib vaccine was distributed, countries such as the USA had long since maintained good hygienic practices, with ready access to clean water and antibiotics. Yet the United States experienced rapid declines in cases of the malady following the distribution of the Hib vaccine.[53] There were no significant changes in sanitation, hygiene, and nutrition to contribute to this outcome. Additionally, the resurgence of measles in countries with good hygienic practices and sanitation, including the US and the UK, further demonstrate the need for vaccines despite excellent living conditions. Such outbreaks can be traced back to under-vaccinated populations, rather than any changes in hygienic conditions, sanitation, or nutritional factors.

Finally, it should be remembered that antibiotics treat diseases caused by bacteria, but not those resulting from viral pathogens. It is also the case that while sanitation can decrease the rates of diseases spread primarily through food or water, like diarrheal diseases, these measures have minimal effects on diseases that are hosted in humans. For instance, pathogens such as hepatitis B, measles, and polio can be spread from person-to-person, as well as through the air. As a result, sanitation is simply not enough to stop their spread, and vaccines are needed to do the heavy lifting of disease control. Plus, in relation to the next myth, this heavy lifting is preferrable to the seeming benefits of natural infection.

Myth #4: Natural immunity is better than vaccinating

It is not unusual for people to express wariness about vaccines, because they are thought to be unnatural. Such views can be linked to what can be described as the *naturalistic heuristic*, which overlaps with health intuitions (Chapter 2). This heuristic is an often deeply held, and reflexive conviction that what is natural is better than what is unnatural.[54] Counter-vaccine media frequently articulates this bias by portraying vaccination as an unnatural procedure, while describing vaccines as being filled with dangerous chemicals and toxic ingredients.[55] In concert with such claims, natural immunity gained from getting infected by a disease is depicted as being superior to the artificial immunity derived from unnatural, human-synthesised injections. The vital question to answer then, is whether natural immunity truly is better than getting vaccinated?

It is important to recall that destroyed or weakened naturally occurring pathogens are one of the primary ingredients of most vaccines (Chapter 1). When a vaccine is injected into a patient's body, it triggers the individual's natural in-built immune mechanisms and teaches the body how to fend off disease. At its core, vaccination is predicated upon the natural functions of human physiology, and vaccines are derived around elements related to natural pathogens. Furthermore, many of the so-called "chemical" ingredients in vaccines occur naturally in the world around us. For example, formaldehyde is sometimes used for the production of vaccines in order to detoxify bacterial toxins or to inactivate viruses.[56] Consequently, residual amounts of formaldehyde can be found in certain vaccines. While this might sound ominous, in "most organisms, including humans, naturally produced formaldehyde is physiologically present as a metabolic byproduct in all bodily fluids, cells, and tissues."[57] Formaldehyde is a necessary component of human cell metabolism, and it occurs naturally in our bodies (Chapter 4).

Determining what is natural and unnatural, therefore, can be far more complicated than what people's naturalistic heuristic reactions might first lead them to believe. At the same time, it is also the case that many things that are natural are not in fact good for us. Snake venom, for instance, is 100% natural, but it can certainly kill you. Similar complexity applies to questions of whether natural immunity is better than the immunological protection afforded to us by vaccines. It is true that natural infections can often result in more robust immunity when compared to vaccines. For this reason, numerous vaccines require several doses to ensure long-term protection. A single shot does not always elicit a sufficient immune response the first time around. Conversely, the disadvantage of natural infection is that it requires individuals to potentially suffer through the full spectrum of symptoms that a disease may inflict, which is exactly what vaccines are designed to avoid. For measles, which is not always regarded as a threatening disease, this means that gaining natural immunity involves the risk of a 1 in 500 chance of death, along with other morbidities.[58] On the other hand, the chances of experiencing a severe response to the MMR vaccine, such as an acute allergic reaction, would be 0.00716% per dose.[59] So natural immunity might be more robust, but the price paid for gaining it in any given population would be incredibly high when compared to the safety of the immunity induced by vaccines.

Along with the 1:500 chance of death resulting from measles, natural infections from diseases that are frequently considered to be relatively benign would also result in widespread infirmities. Approximately 1 in every 1,000 children who contract Chickenpox (varicella) develop "severe pneumonia (infection of the lungs) or encephalitis (infection of the brain)."[60] Furthermore, about "1 of every 50 women infected with varicella during their pregnancy will deliver children with birth defects."[61] These birth defects "include developmental delay and shortened or atrophied limbs."[62] In children who contract Haemophilus Influenzae Type B (Hib), a bacterium that can infect the lining of the brain and cause meningitis, approximately 3% to 6% die.[63] Up to 30% of people who recover from Hib, and gain natural immunity from it, are left with permanent neurological sequalae. Neurological sequelae are "focal neurological deficits, hearing loss, cognitive impairment and epilepsy."[64]

The serious side effects and death statistics that accompany gaining natural immunity from vaccine preventable diseases are substantial. Yet the immunity derived from vaccines does not extract such a severe price. In that respect, natural immunity is patently not better than immunity achieved through vaccination. It is also the case that a handful of vaccines can trigger *better* immune responses than are usually derived from natural infections. These include immunological results from the Hib vaccine, the human papillomavirus (HPV) vaccine, the pneumococcal vaccine, and the tetanus shot.[65] This reveals that while vaccines have been described as an unnatural procedure, inferior to natural infection, the scientific data and stats say otherwise. The problem, of course, is that facts are not necessarily convincing. Plus, in tandem with Distrust statements, the Confidence theme encourages individuals to put trust in facts and sources other than those conforming with the scientific consensus on vaccines.

Considering Confidence and consensus

When it comes to vaccination choices, and the DCD of antivaccine communications, it is the Confidence theme that attempts to answer the following question for audiences: Who can you really trust? Confidence messaging is the converse of Distrust in counter-vaccination messaging. Where Distrust is concentrated upon increasing scepticism towards vaccines and scientific experts, the Confidence theme fills the trust gap by instructing people about who they can really rely on instead of the scientific consensus and leading medical authorities. Confidence features claims of expertise, as well as techniques that can be employed for building credibility and demonstrating trustworthiness. In antivaccination messages this can include references to the purported academic degrees and scientific training of vaccine-sceptical experts. Counter-immunisation media can frequently refer to a handful of antivaccination specialists who are apparently highly trained scientists, or medical practitioners, opposed to vaccines.

In relation to such claims, it is vital to note is that there is strong scientific consensus from the world's experts regarding the safety and efficacy of vaccines. Along with other leading institutions, the Centers for Disease Control and Prevention, the National Academies of Sciences, Engineering, and Medicine, the National Institutes of Health, and the World Health Organization collectively validate that vaccines are safe and effective.[66] In fact, as one study found, this consensus is so firm that a majority of scientists in the American Association for the Advancement of Science also stated that vaccines should be compulsory for all children.[67] In regard to this scientific agreement, studies have indicated that intentionally drawing attention to the significant degree of medical consensus about vaccine safety maintained by experts can help increase public support for vaccines.[68] One report found that when participants were told that "90% of medical scientists agree that childhood vaccines are safe, this not only increased people's intention to vaccinate their children," but it also "lowered perceptions of vaccine risk, and helped to correct 'sticky' misperceptions," including the false "belief that vaccines cause autism."[69]

Nevertheless, identifying a handful of apparent vaccine-sceptical experts, with seemingly legitimate credentials, can amplify the perceived significance of contrarian views. This might make it appear as though there is more disagreement about vaccine science than there truthfully is. It also provides the antivaccination movement with the persuasive appearance of being endorsed by genuine experts. The difficulty is that even though thousands upon thousands of researchers, leading scientific institutions, and reams of empirical data together support the safety and effectiveness of vaccines, a small group of professed scientists, from official sounding organisations, can still be convincing to audiences. Along with touting antivaccine experts, the Confidence theme can further involve highlighting the credentials of pro-vaccine authorities when it is beneficial to do so. For example, some pro-vaccine academics have questioned the fairness of mandatory and punitive vaccination policies, even though these individuals fully support society-wide vaccination efforts. Counter-vaccination media can seize upon these critiques, emphasising that such credentialed researchers appear to support antivaccination opposition to compulsory vaccination.[70]

Besides referring to specialists, Confidence-related messages may also feature reports about the personal expertise maintained by vaccine-sceptical parents and antivaccination leaders. These statements can include references to professional training, which is usually not related to vaccine development or affiliated medical fields. Yet these proficiencies are used to serve as an individual's proof of intellect and ability. Accordingly, even though anti-vaccination media makers are frequently not scientific experts, they can often refer to their own university-level education, while claiming to have completed extensive research online and in academic peer-reviewed litera-ture. Along with such markers of personal expertise, counter-vaccine mes-sages often point to the credibility of past experiences, including allegations of having had direct, firsthand exposure to vaccine caused injuries or death. Antivaccine messages can also imply that vaccine-hesitant individuals, who do their own research, are in fact *more* informed than pro-vaccination authorities and doctors.[71]

At the same time, the Confidence theme can involve more general references to scientific evidence and data that are said to substantiate vac-cine-scepticism. Audiences are frequently told that antivaccination views are backed up by real science, including peer reviewed research and empirical facts. Additionally, antivaccine messages can refer the sheer number of people who are also doubtful of vaccinations. This conveys to audiences that they can have confidence in the fact that they are not the only ones who might be experiencing vaccine hesitancy. This may involve mentioning how many individuals around the world claim to have been negatively affected by vaccines, while affirming that an important number of other people might also have grave concerns over vaccine safety. Sometimes these messages can feature statistics to demonstrate the percentages of people, including even medical professionals, who apparently have doubts, or who have had firsthand experiences with vaccine injuries.[72]

For all these reasons, the Confidence theme delivers assurances to audiences that they are not alone in their misgivings, while insisting that anti-vaccination claims are supported by scientific experts, empirical research, and personal experiences. This theme is important to understand because when it comes to scientific topics such as vaccination, the general public often relies upon expert opinions to help shape their own positions. While Distrust narratives actively question consensus science, Confidence messaging is how antivaccine arguments garner the appearance of credibility to influence hesitant audiences. The theme is also strongly associated with several persuasive cues, and one fundamental vaccine myth. This myth relates that an abundance of both evidence and experts dispute the definitive scientific consensus around vaccines.[73]

Myth #5: Research and experts discredit the scientific consensus

The Confidence theme of antivaccination communications is based upon claims that there are numerous specialists and credible data that challenge the scientific verdict on vaccines. Confidence messages also include assertions from non-experts about how much research they themselves have conducted. The premise of such statements is that a small number of experts discredit the consensus, while affirming that vaccine-sceptics can be far more knowledgeable than trained specialists. Such claims can be particularly irksome for medical practitioners. As Maya J. Goldenberg has observed, this is because healthcare works recognise that the scientific consensus is "overwhelmingly supportive of childhood vaccination as a safe and effective means of preventing serious illness."[74]

Selectivity and the consilience of evidence

Goldenberg's remark stands out because a central characteristic of ardent vaccine denial is the rejection of this scientific consensus. In fact, refusing to accept academic consensus appears to be a common feature of science denialism; whether it involves rejecting human caused climate change, the fact that HIV causes AIDS, or the safety and effectiveness of vaccines.[75] As Diethelm and Mckee have explained, in all such cases:

> There is an overwhelming consensus on the evidence among scientists yet there are also vocal commentators who reject this consensus,

convincing many of the public, and often the media too, that the consensus is not based on "sound science" or denying that there is a consensus by exhibiting individual dissenting voices as the ultimate authorities on the topic in question. Their goal is to convince that there are sufficient grounds to reject the case for taking action to tackle threats to health.[76]

To persuade audiences that there are good reasons for rejecting the consensus, science deniers employ *selectivity*. Selectivity involves "drawing on isolated papers that challenge the dominant consensus or highlighting the flaws in the weakest papers among those that support it as a means of discrediting the entire field."[77]

In the case of the antivaccination movement, the quintessential example of such selectivity in action includes ongoing references to a 1998 paper in the journal *Lancet*. This paper posited a theoretical link between the Measles, Mumps, Rubella vaccine, chronic inflammation of the digestive tract, and the development of autism.[78] The paper was based on observations of only 12 children, and 10 of the article's 13 authors later retracted the study. The retraction stated, "We wish to make it clear that in this paper no causal link was established between MMR vaccine and autism as the data were insufficient."[79] Since the publication of this withdrawn article, at least 27 studies conducted around the world have refuted claims that the MMR vaccine is connected to autism.[80] In 2010, the United States Court of Federal Claims also adjudicated over more than 5,000 cases that claimed vaccines had caused autism in children. The proceedings found that there was no evidence to support a link between autism and vaccines, despite the hearings being criticized "for having an overly permissive evidentiary test for causation and for granting credence to insupportable accusations of vaccine harm."[81] That is to say, even though the hearings permitted claimants to enter "scientific evidence and testimony that would likely be inadmissible" in other courts, the judges *still* ruled that there was no evidential foundation to allegations that vaccines cause autism.[82]

Andrew Wakefield was "found guilty of serious professional misconduct and struck off the medical register by the General Medical Council," and the *Lancet* article has been described as "one of the most serious frauds in medical history."[83] Nevertheless, the 1998 paper and Wakefield are still lauded as confirmation that vaccinations lead to autism. The central problem with such selectivity is that it ignores the vast majority of experts, and the preponderance of data refuting antivaccination claims. Selectivity also operates under the false assumption that finding a few studies, and having a handful of purported experts onside, discredits consensus science. This is not the way that science functions. Scientific consensus results from the accumulation of research findings, corroborated independently by different researchers over time, which are accepted by a majority of experts. This involves a consensus of knowledge acquired through the *consilience of evidence*. A consilience of evidence occurs when "the consensus is based on varied lines of evidence that all seem to agree with each other."[84] This requires that different varieties of separately sourced data all match up and point to the same conclusions. Scientific consensus develops when the bulk of specialists agree, and this accord is established by the unanimity of research findings, reported across a range of studies. The agreement arises from diverse types of data, amassed in peer-reviewed scientific literature, which end up telling the same story.[85] Even if a few studies, or a small number of experts disagree with the scientific consensus, it does not follow that the consensus is in jeopardy. This is because a handful of contrarian studies likely do not demonstrate a consilience of evidence.

It may still be the case that having a few studies, or several specialists with impressive degrees onboard to confirm antivaccination views is convincing. Even so, when the vast majority of experts and peer reviewed articles diverge with what a small number of contrarian studies and specialists are saying, it is a signal to be cautious about their claims. In fact, if a movement employs selectivity, this should serve as a warning that what the group endorses is likely faulty. This is because selectivity demonstrates that allegations are not supported by the weight of scientific data. A lack of academic support forces science deniers, including vaccine-sceptics, to look to a handful of supportive experts and studies that do not maintain a consilience of evidence, and which are rejected by the majority of specialists. Such science denying authorities have been described as "fake experts," who are "individuals who purport to be experts in a particular area but whose views are entirely inconsistent with established knowledge."[86] It is for these reasons that anti-vaccination media makers are compelled to refer to a relatively small pool of studies and experts, including Wakefield's 1998 debunked study, instead of the preponderance of research that has long since falsified it.

Doing your own research does not make you a true expert

It is not uncommon for antivaccination media to claim that vaccine-hesitant parents are *more* informed than pro-vaccination authorities.[87] For instance, a counter-vaccine commentator has asserted that "parents who have studied the issue of vaccination by reading medical journal articles and texts and by speaking with a broad range of health professionals can be far more knowledgeable about this topic than the average GP."[88] The message is that non-expert individuals, who do their own research into vaccination, can be as informed, or even more so, than highly trained medical practitioners. The problem is simply that doing one's own research is not going to provide the same level of knowledge, practical training, and expertise that medical specialists and scientific researchers obtain through years of dedicated study and hands-on practice.

When I teach university students on this topic, I often refer to my own experiences as a Canadian migrant in Australia, who has been involved with my children's Australian rules football teams. I know the sport's general rules, I watch professional games, and I even read up online about what is happening throughout the season. Yet as a Canadian who migrated to Australia's fair shores, I have never actually played a game of Aussie rules football. Consequently, while I have conducted what might seem like substantial online research about the sport from home, gone to numerous games as a fan, and learned enough about the basics to teach youngsters on the field, I still cannot be trusted over the paid athletes to kick a goal during a professional game. I also could not be relied upon to successfully coach a professional team to victory. The best people to have on the field and coach are sportspersons with years of experience playing and coaching at the highest levels. This same premise is true when it comes to science and medicine, but science and medicine are far more complicated and difficult to understand than Australian rules football. It is important, therefore, that we put our trust in people who are reputable, and that we rely on experts who have the educational backgrounds, necessary training, and practical experience truly needed to speak with confidence about vaccines. This is why it is also necessary to be cautious about claims that someone is more knowledgeable about vaccines than trained experts. Without years of dedicated medical and scientific training, such individuals cannot be relied upon to make accurate verdicts about vaccine safety and effectiveness.

Confidence and Source Cues

A central feature of the Confidence theme are references to antivaccine medical specialists and empirical evidence, including remarks about the professional training, university education, and past experiences of vaccine hesitant individuals. Such mentions can occur in personal narratives about vaccine doubt. As noted above, these accounts frequently incorporate claims of having done extensive research into vaccines to discover significant amounts of data to warrant vaccine-scepticism. In this vein, for example, one individual who described herself as an occupational therapist explained online that there is "ample scientific evidence that I have available to me as a health practitioner to support my choice as a parent not to vaccinate my children."[89] These sorts of references to expertise and scientific evidence are associated with the persuasive cue described as *Source Cues*.[90]

In situations of low elaboration likelihood, where there is a lack of motivation or ability to meticulously investigate a communication's claims, the alleged expertise and perceived credibility of communicators has been demonstrated to act as a significant peripheral cue.[91] "Sources who are credible are ones with superior knowledge (expertise)" and this apparent knowledge is often relied upon when people decide to accept or reject persuasive messages.[92] If the same individual presents an identical message to different groups of people, the message's persuasive arguments are accepted far more readily by audiences who have been told that the speaker holds academic credentials from a prestigious university.[93] Credibility can also be increased through certain attire, such as a uniform or lab coat, and even the presence of specific scientific equipment, such as microscopes and test tubes, can generate scientific authority and credibility. Statements professing that scientific data or evidence support a position can also be similarly used to cultivate this persuasive technique. Correspondingly, credibility is a function of the messenger's supposed trustworthiness, objectivity, and personal confidence, while societal status and prestige can further cultivate estimations of expertise.[94] This is why celebrity spokespeople can also serve as persuasive representatives who are often featured in advertising, simply due to their societal status and public prominence.[95] It may also be why celebrities supporting antivaccination messages appear to be particularly influential for audiences who are more enamoured by celebrity actors, athletes and influencers.[96]

Source Cues, therefore, can be identified as displays of academic qualifications, expertise, references to scientific data and empirical evidence, as well as appeals to celebrity. In antivaccination media, Source Cues signal to audiences that counter-vaccine sources are trustworthy and can be relied upon when making vaccine decisions.[97] It is important to be aware of such claims, because reports about expertise can legitimise counter-vaccine views to audiences and help secure the perception that an antivaccination stance is supported by scientific findings, some medical professionals, and numerous scientific experts.[98]

Social Consensus and the Confidence theme

While antivaccination messages regularly defy the scientific consensus, the Confidence theme also consists of appeals to social agreement. This includes referring to the large number of other people who also have vaccine hesitancy, or who claim to have experienced vaccine caused injuries.[99] Even though antivaccination is not supported by the weight of data and scientific consensus, counter-vaccine messages often allude to the sheer quantity of individuals who are likeminded in their distrust of vaccination. Alternatively, counter-vaccine media sometimes portrays antivaccinationists as a brave minority of individuals who are valiantly fighting against the ruling elite.[100] In such cases, vaccine sceptics are presented as a heroic band of "fighters who never give up no matter how much the government and vested pharmaceutical interests want us to."[101] Altogether, suggestions that an important quantity of people endorse a marketed product, or an advertised opinion coincide with the persuasive cue defined as *Social Consensus*.[102]

Multiple sources, social proof, and underdog effects

On the whole, Social Consensus is a persuasive lever hinged upon the tendency of people to follow the *herd*, as it harnesses the drive to imitate or conform to the social behaviours of those around us. One aspect of this psychological phenomenon is the common inclination to give more weight to ideas that are stated by multiple sources. In fact, studies have indicated that hearing the same or similar messages from more than one source increases the processing of communications by audiences, and it can also serve as a peripheral cue in low elaboration likelihood contexts.[103] Though it is not understood exactly why listening to matching statements from several different sources influences persuasion, Petty and Cacioppo have explained that when elaboration likelihood is low, audiences "may use the number of people who support the issue as a simple cue as to the worth of the proposal."[104] That is, people seem more likely to agree with a message stated by several different voices because it appears to reflect a type of social agreement.

Source Consensus also includes appeals to social proof, which involves highlighting the beliefs, behaviours, and testimonials of others for persuasion purposes. Social proof can be influential because individuals are inclined to "use the opinions apparently held in their immediate social context to form judgments."[105] People also "tend to align their beliefs with the opinions of those around them."[106] Accordingly, persuasive communicators are not, by necessity, required to convince audiences that an idea deserves reception, but simply that many other people believe that it does. Appeals to social proof can generate long-lasting opinions and serve as peripheral cues, especially when individuals are unfamiliar with information and unsure about how to act.[107] Advertising testimonials from satisfied customers function in this manner, as do public opinion polls associated with the use of statistics, which can cause an audience to shift personal attitudes to coincide with majority positions.[108] Additionally, if message recipients exhibiting low elaboration likelihood simply hear a positive audience reaction to a communication, such as applause, it tends to cause the message to be perceived as being more persuasive.[109] Social proof also does not necessarily need to appeal to the largest population groups in a society, but can refer to a majority of individuals in the specific community that a communicator is attempting to influence.

Another subcategory of Social Consensus includes underdog effects, which involves purposefully stressing the seemingly underdog nature of an idea, action, or group. An underdog can be described as anything, or any persons expected to lose a contest due to a lack of ability or popularity or if they are the victim of some form of injustice. For persuasion purposes, such an underdog group may be characterised as a band of righteous dissenters or victims, contesting against a domineering, and even deceitful majority or group of elites that is conspiring against them. Accordingly, instead of being asked to join the majority, an audience is rallied to enlist with a seemingly noble minority social consensus. Underdog effects are often less predictable than are appeals to social proof, though appealing to the underdog can still prove influential. In particular, underdog claims appear most effective when elaboration likelihood can be described as being low due to a lack of information available to an audience, or when listeners are somewhat indifferent to the ideas being presented in a communication.[110]

Confidence, statistics and jargon

Along with referencing public consensus and expertise, antivaccination media sometimes feature poll results in combination with particular statistics. These are frequently used to demonstrate the number of people, including medical professionals, who apparently have vaccination doubts, or who have firsthand experience with vaccine injuries. In relation to the Confidence theme, such numbers assure audiences that many other laypeople and medical professionals also have vaccine uncertainties.[111] Accordingly, an online post discussed a journal article which apparently "shows that a large number of nurses (98% of them surveyed) – people who are trained to understand how vaccines are meant to work and how safe they are purported to be – are saying no to vaccination."[112] Notably, the use of such questionable statistics in antivaccination media, as well as complex scientific language, together express characteristics associated with the persuasive cue described as *Statistics and Technical Jargon*.[113]

Robert Levine has explained that when a message includes statistics, these numbers can serve as a marker of expertise "even when they're meaningless."[114] Statistics can persuasively signal a communicator's know-how by making use of people's *innumeracy*. This innumeracy has been described as an audience's "functional incompetence to understand and argue back to a statistic, and to draw accurate meaning from, and criticize, a statistical argument about the real world."[115] An audience's inability to fully grasp the statistical information can then lead individuals to peripherally depend on other evidence that points to whether the communicator is a credible source. As one study concluded, statistics were found to cause people "to rely on a peripheral cue – the character of the communicator – as a basis for judgment, so that an expert communicator induced greater persuasion than did a source of lower expertise."[116] In antivaccine messages, dubious statistics can be employed to substantiate claims about vaccine ineffectiveness, and to demonstrate that vaccines are mathematically confirmed to be dangerous.[117]

The use of technical jargon in media seems to operate in a similar persuasive manner as do statistics. Technical jargon is complex language that may be incomprehensible to non-specialists. As with statistical information, studies suggest that there is a complementary relationship between the use of complicated jargon and the perceived expertise of a communicator. For instance, when a communicator uses highly specialized scientific terms, audiences tend to rely on the presenter's credentials to determine the persuasiveness of the message. If both jargon and credentials are presented to audiences, a message is more frequently judged to be convincing. However, if jargon is not complemented with impressive credentials, then such complex language is thought to be less compelling. In this sense, jargon triggers persuasion via Source Cues, while it is also dependent upon them.[118] Technical jargon is a regular feature of online counter-vaccine articles, which employ complex chemical terminology to discuss vaccine ingredients and unproven autism–vaccine links.[119]

Confidence, Distrust and counter-vaccine persuasion

Altogether then, it is important to be mindful of how different kinds of jargon and statistics are being used in antivaccination messages. It is also worth remembering that statistics and technical jargon are most persuasive when they are employed alongside references to a communicator's expertise and credibility. These cues are also part and parcel of the Distrust and Confidence themes in counter-vaccine arguments. Overall, Distrust communicates that people's health choices are being restricted by undemocratic and untrustworthy governments, working in collusion with BigPharma. At the same, Distrust messaging relates that counter-vaccine data and immunisation injury reports are being suppressed worldwide. The Confidence theme counterbalances such Distrust messaging, by emphasising the personal expertise of sceptical individuals, the credentials of specialists as well as the science behind antivaccination claims. It also features the numbers of other, often similarly experienced people who also support counter-vaccine initiatives. In this way, the Confidence theme underlines who and what data audiences can be confident in.

Notes

1 Jinxuan Ma and Lynne Stahl, "A Multimodal Critical Discourse Analysis of Anti-Vaccination Information on Facebook," *Library and Information Science Research* 39, no. 4 (2017): 304; Jeanette B. Ruiz and Robert A. Bell, "Understanding Vaccination Resistance: Vaccine Search Term Selection Bias and the Valence of Retrieved Information," *Vaccine* 32, no. 44 (2014); Meghan Bridgid Moran et al., "What Makes Anti-Vaccine Websites Persuasive? A Content Analysis of Techniques Used by Anti-Vaccine Websites to Engender Anti-Vaccine Sentiment," *Journal of Communication in Healthcare* 9, no. 3 (2016); Thomas Aechtner, "Distrust, Danger, and Confidence: A Content Analysis of the Australian Vaccination-Risks Network Blog," *Public Understanding of Science* (2020).

2 Katie Attwell et al., "Vaccine Rejecting Parents' Engagement with Expert Systems That Inform Vaccination Programs," *Bioethical Inquiry* 14, no. 1 (2017); Thomas Aechtner and Jeremy Farr, "Religion, Trust, and Vaccine Hesitancy in Australia: An Examination of Two Surveys," *Journal for the Academic Study of Religion* 35, no. 2 (2022); Charlotte Lee et al., "Hurdles to Herd Immunity: Distrust of Government and Vaccine Refusal in the US, 2002–2003," *Vaccine* 34, no. 34 (2016); Radomír Masaryk and Mária Hatoková, "Qualitative Inquiry into Reasons Why Vaccination Messages Fail," *Journal of Health Psychology* 22, no. 14 (2017): 6–7; Heidi J. Larson et al., "Addressing

the Vaccine Confidence Gap," *Lancet* 378, no. 9790 (2011); Attwell et al., "Vaccine Rejecting Parents' Engagement with Expert Systems That Inform Vaccination Programs"; Jeffrey V. Lazarus et al., "A Global Survey of Potential Acceptance of a COVID-19 Vaccine," *Nature Medicine* 27, no. 2 (2021); Jeffrey V. Lazarus et al., "Revisiting COVID-19 Vaccine Hesitancy around the World Using Data from 23 Countries in 2021," *Nature Communications* 13, no. 1 (2022); Paul R. Ward et al., "Understanding the Perceived Logic of Care by Vaccine-Hesitant and Vaccine-Refusing Parents: A Qualitative Study in Australia," *PLoS One* 12, no. 10 (2017); Ohid Yaqub et al., "Attitudes to Vaccination: A Critical Review," *Social Science & Medicine* 112 (2014).

3   Dhamanpreet Dhaliwal and Cynthia Mannion, "Antivaccine Messages on Facebook: Preliminary Audit," *JMIR Public Health and Surveillance* 6, no. 4 (2020); Kate Faasse, Casey J. Chatman, and Leslie R. Martin, "A Comparison of Language Use in Pro- and Anti-Vaccination Comments in Response to a High Profile Facebook Post," *Vaccine* 34, no. 47 (2016); Naomi Smith and Tim Graham, "Mapping the Anti-Vaccination Movement on Facebook," *Information, Communication & Society* 22, no. 9 (2019).

4   Ward et al., "Understanding the Perceived Logic of Care by Vaccine-Hesitant and Vaccine-Refusing Parents: A Qualitative Study in Australia," 13.

5   Choudhary Sobhan Shakeel et al., "Global COVID-19 Vaccine Acceptance: A Systematic Review of Associated Social and Behavioral Factors," *Vaccines* 10, no. 1 (2022).

6   Cass R. Sunstein and Adrian Vermeule, "Conspiracy Theories: Causes and Cures," *Journal of Political Philosophy* 17, no. 2 (2009): 205.

7   Aechtner, "Distrust, Danger, and Confidence: A Content Analysis of the Australian Vaccination-Risks Network Blog."

8   Brian Hughes et al., "Development of a Codebook of Online Anti-Vaccination Rhetoric to Manage COVID-19 Vaccine Misinformation," *International Journal of Environmental Research and Public Health* 18, no. 14 (2021).

9   Aechtner, "Distrust, Danger, and Confidence: A Content Analysis of the Australian Vaccination-Risks Network Blog."

10 Jennifer A. Whitson and Adam D. Galinsky, "Lacking Control Increases Illusory Pattern Perception," *Science* 322, no. 5898 (2008); Ray Pratt, "Theorizing Conspiracy," *Theory and Society* 32, no. 2 (2003).

11 Jan-Willem van Prooijen and Karen M. Douglas, "Conspiracy Theories as Part of History: The Role of Societal Crisis Situations," *Memory Studies* 10, no. 3 (2017): 329.

12 Victoria Emma Pagán, *Conspiracy Theory in Latin Literature* (Austin: University of Texas Press, 2012), 5.

13 Viren Swami and Adrian Furnham, "Political Paranoia and Conspiracy Theories," in *Power, Politics, and Paranoia: Why People Are Suspicious About Their Leaders*, ed. Jan-Willem van Prooijen and Paul A. M. Van Lange (Cambridge: Cambridge University Press, 2012).

14 Viren Swami et al., "Conspiracist Ideation in Britain and Austria: Evidence of a Monological Belief System and Associations between Individual Psychological Differences and Real-World and Fictitious Conspiracy Theories," *British Journal of Psychology* 102, no. 3 (2011): 444.

15 Mikey Biddlestone et al., "Conspiracy Beliefs and the Individual, Relational, and Collective Selves," *Social and Personality Psychology Compass* 15, no. 10 (2021).

16 Marta Marchlewska et al., "From Bad to Worse: Avoidance Coping with Stress Increases Conspiracy Beliefs," *Br J Soc Psychol* 61, no. 2 (2022); Jais Adam-Troian et al., "Of Precarity and Conspiracy: Introducing a Socio-Functional Model of Conspiracy Beliefs," *British Journal of Social Psychology* (2022).

17 Viren Swami et al., "Analytic Thinking Reduces Belief in Conspiracy Theories," *Cognition* 133, no. 3 (2014).

18 Valerie van Mulukom et al., "Antecedents and Consequences of COVID-19 Conspiracy Beliefs: A Systematic Review," *Social Science & Medicine* 301 (2022); Pascal Wagner-Egger et al., "The Yellow Vests in France: Psychosocial Determinants and Consequences of the Adherence to a Social Movement in a Representative Sample of the Population," *International Review of Social Psychology* 35, no. 1 (2022).

19 Anthony Lantian et al., "'I Know Things They Don't Know!': The Role of Need for Uniqueness in Belief in Conspiracy Theories," *Social Psychology* 48, no. 3 (2017).

20 Aechtner, "Distrust, Danger, and Confidence: A Content Analysis of the Australian Vaccination-Risks Network Blog"; Moran et al., "What Makes Anti-Vaccine Websites Persuasive? A Content Analysis of Techniques Used by Anti-Vaccine Websites to Engender Anti-Vaccine Sentiment."

21 Paul Ward, "To Trust or Not to Trust (in Doctors)? That Is the Question," *Archives of Disease in Childhood* 103, no. 8 (2018): 718.

22 Gilla K. Shapiro et al., "Validation of the Vaccine Conspiracy Beliefs Scale," *Papillomavirus Research* 2 (2016): 167.

23 David Robert Grimes, "On the Viability of Conspiratorial Beliefs. (Report)," *Plos One* 11, no. 1 (2016): 2.

24 Stephane A. Rngnier and Jasper Huels, "Drug Versus Vaccine Investment: A Modelled Comparison of Economic Incentives. (Report)," *Cost Effectiveness and Resource Allocation* 11, no. 23 (2013): 1.

25 "Vaccine Myth: Vaccines are Just Money-Makers for Big Pharma & Doctors," *Boost Oregon*, https://www.boostoregon.org/blog/vaccine-myth-vaccines-a re-just-moneymakers-for-big-pharma-and-doctors.

26 Judith E. Glazner, Brenda Beaty, and Stephen Berman, "Cost of Vaccine Administration among Pediatric Practices," *Pediatrics* 124, no. Supplement (2009).

27 Judith E. Glazner et al., "The Cost of Giving Childhood Vaccinations: Differences among Provider Types," *Pediatrics* 113, no. 6 (2004); Courtney A. Gidengil et al., "Financial Barriers to the Adoption of Combination Vaccines by Pediatricians," *Archives of Pediatrics & Adolescent Medicine* 164, no. 12 (2010).

28 Margaret S. Coleman et al., "Net Financial Gain or Loss from Vaccination in Pediatric Medical Practices," *Pediatrics* 124, no. 5 (2009): S472.

29 "Catch-up Incentives for Vaccination Providers Fact Sheet," Australian Government: Department of Health, https://www.health.gov.au/sites/default/files/catchup-incentives-vaccination-providers.pdf.

30 Meryl Dorey, "Vaccination and Health – Your Right to Choose Seminars Western Nsw-August 2012," AVN, https://avn.org.au/2012/06/vaccina tion-and-health-your-right-to-choose-seminars-western-nsw-august-2012/.

31 Robert B. Cialdini, *Influence: Science and Practice*, 5th ed. (Boston: Pearson Education, 2009), 204.

32 Stephen Worchel, Jerry Lee, and Akanbi Adewole, "Effects of Supply and Demand on Ratings of Object Value," *Journal of Personality and Social Psychology* 32, no. 5 (1975); Michael Lynn, "Scarcity Effects on Value: A Quantitative Review of the Commodity Theory Literature," *Psychology & Marketing* 8, no. 1 (1991); Michael Lynn and Paulette Bogert, "The Effect of Scarcity on Anticipated Price Appreciation," *Journal of Applied Social Psychology* 26, no. 22 (1996).

33 "Cross-National Differences in Proneness to Scarcity Effects: The Moderating Roles of Familiarity, Uncertainty Avoidance, and Need for Cognitive Closure," *Psychology & Marketing* 21, no. 9 (2004): 740.

34 Stephen Worchel, Susan Arnold, and Michael Baker, "The Effects of Censorship and Attractiveness of the Censor on Attitude Change," *Journal of Applied Social Psychology* 5, no. 3 (1975).

35 Sharon S. Brehm and Jack W. Brehm, *Psychological Reactance: A Theory of Freedom and Control* (New York: Academic Press, 1981), 108.

36 Jack W. Brehm et al., "The Attractiveness of an Eliminated Choice Alternative," *Journal of Experimental Social Psychology* 2, no. 3 (1966).

37 Sharon Wolf and David A. Montgomery, "Effects of Inadmissible Evidence and Level of Judicial Admonishment to Disregard on the Judgments of Mock Jurors," *Journal of Applied Social Psychology* 7, no. 3 (1977).

38 Meryl Dorey, "Nurses Don't Trust Vaccines," AVN, https://avn.org.au/2012/04/nurses-dont-trust-vaccines/.

39 Aechtner, "Distrust, Danger, and Confidence: A Content Analysis of the Australian Vaccination-Risks Network Blog."

40 Hatoková, "Qualitative Inquiry into Reasons Why Vaccination Messages Fail," 7.

41 "Measles Elimination," Centers for Disease Control and Prevention, https://www.cdc.gov/measles/elimination.html.

42 "Measles Vaccine: Canadian Immunization Guide," Government of Canada, https://www.canada.ca/en/public-health/services/publications/healthy-living/canadian-immunization-guide-part-4-active-vaccines/page-12-measles-vaccine.html; Aechtner, "Distrust, Danger, and Confidence: A Content Analysis of the Australian Vaccination-Risks Network Blog."

43 "Measles," Centers for Disease Control and Prevention, https://www.cdc.gov/vaccines/pubs/pinkbook/meas.html.

44 "More Than 140,000 Die from Measles as Cases Surge Worldwide," World Health Organization, https://www.who.int/news-room/detail/05-12-2019-more-than-140-000-die-from-measles-as-cases-surge-worldwide.

45 Ibid.

46 Ibid.

47 K. Alexander, M. Wickens, and S. M. Fletcher-Lartey, "Measles Elimination in Australia," *Australian Journal of General Practice* 49, no. 3 (2020): 112.

48 Ibid.

49 Lucija Tomljenovic, "Forced Vaccinations: For the Greater Good?," *The Vaccine Choice Journal* Special Supplement (2015): 8.

50 Kenneth A. Reinert, *No Small Hope: Towards the Universal Provision of Basic Goods* (New York: Oxford University Press, 2018).

51 "Goal 6: Ensure Access to Water and Sanitation for All," United Nations, https://www.un.org/sustainabledevelopment/water-and-sanitation/.

52 Reinert, *No Small Hope: Towards the Universal Provision of Basic Goods.*

53 "Haemophilus Influenzae Type B," Centers for Disease Control, https://www.cdc.gov/vaccines/pubs/pinkbook/hib.html; "3. Who Benefits from Vaccines?," Australian Academy of Science, https://www.science.org.au/learning/general-audience/science-booklets/science-immunisation/3-who-benefits-vaccines.

54 Tara C. Smith, "Vaccine Rejection and Hesitancy: A Review and Call to Action," *Open Forum Infectious Diseases* 4, no. 3 (2017): 1; A. Reich Jennifer, *Calling the Shots* (New York: New York University Press, 2016), 116.

55 Tomljenovic, "Forced Vaccinations: For the Greater Good?."

56 Robert J. Mitkus, Maureen A. Hess, and Sorell L. Schwartz, "Pharmacokinetic Modeling as an Approach to Assessing the Safety of Residual Formaldehyde in Infant Vaccines," *Vaccine* 31, no. 25 (2013).

57 Luoping Zhang, *Formaldehyde: Exposure, Toxicity and Health Effects* (Cambridge: Royal Society of Chemistry, 2018), 2.

58 "Vaccine Myths Debunked," https://www.publichealth.org/public-awareness/understanding-vaccines/vaccine-myths-debunked/.

59 A. Kalet et al., "Allergic Reactions to MMR Vaccine," *Pediatrics* 89, no. 1 (1992).

60 "A Look at Each Vaccine: Varicella Vaccine," https://www.chop.edu/centers-programs/vaccine-education-center/vaccine-details/varicella-vaccine.

61 Ibid.

62 Ibid.

63 "Haemophilus Influenzae Type B (Hib)," Commonwealth of Australia, https://immunisationhandbook.health.gov.au/vaccine-preventable-diseases/haemophilus-influenzae-type-b-hib.

64 Marjolein J. Lucas, Matthijs C. Brouwer, and Diederik van de Beek, "Neurological Sequelae of Bacterial Meningitis," *The Journal of Infection* 73, no. 1 (2016): 18.

65 "Vaccine Safety: Immune System and Health," Children's Hospital of Philadelphia, https://www.chop.edu/centers-programs/vaccine-education-center/vaccine-safety/immune-system-and-health.

66 "Vaccines and Immunization," World Health Organization, https://www.who.int/health-topics/vaccines-and-immunization#tab=tab_1; "Vaccines & Immunizations," Centers for Disease Control and Prevention, https://www.cdc.gov/vaccines/index.html; Christine Stencel and Luwam Yeibio, "Few Health Problems Are Caused by Vaccines, Iom Report Finds," National Academies of Sciences, Engineering, and Medicine, https://www.nationalacademies.org/news/2011/08/few-health-problems-are-caused-by-vaccines-iom-report-finds; "Vaccines," National Institute of Allergy and Infectious Diseases, https://www.niaid.nih.gov/research/vaccines.

67 Cary Funk et al., *Public and Scientists' Views on Science and Society* (Pew Research Center, 2015), 46.

68 Sander L. van der Linden, Chris E. Clarke, and Edward W. Maibach, "Highlighting Consensus among Medical Scientists Increases Public Support for Vaccines: Evidence from a Randomized Experiment," *BMC Public Health* 15, no. 1 (2015).

69 Sander van Der Linden, "Why Doctors Should Convey the Medical Consensus on Vaccine Safety," *Evidence-Based Medicine* 21, no. 3 (2016): 119.

70 Aechtner, "Distrust, Danger, and Confidence: A Content Analysis of the Australian Vaccination-Risks Network Blog."

71 Ibid., 25.

72 Ibid., 28–29.

73 Philipp Schmid and Noni E. MacDonald, *Best Practice Guidance: How to Respond to Vocal Vaccine Deniers in Public* (Copenhagen: World Health Organization, 2017), 8.

74 "Vaccines, Values and Science," *Canadian Medical Association Journal* 191, no. 14 (2019): E397.

75 Thomas Aechtner, *Media and the Science-Religion Conflict: Mass Persuasion in the Evolution Wars* (Abingdon: Routledge, 2020); "Improving Evolution Advocacy: Translating Vaccine Interventions to the Evolution Wars," *Zygon* 55, no. 1 (2020).

76 Pascal Diethelm and Martin McKee, "Denialism: What Is It and How Should Scientists Respond?," *The European Journal of Public Health* 19, no. 1 (2009): 2.

77 Ibid., 3.

78 A. J. Wakefield et al., "Ileal-Lymphoid-Nodular Hyperplasia, Non-Specific Colitis, and Pervasive Developmental Disorder in Children," *Lancet* 351, no. 9103 (1998).

79   Simon H. Murch et al., "Retraction of an Interpretation," *Lancet* 363, no. 9411 (2004): 750.

80   G. Baird, A. Pickles, and E. Simonoff, "Measles Vaccination and Antibody Response in Autism Spectrum Disorders," *Archives of Disease in Childhood* 93, no. 10 (2008); C. Black, J. Kaye, and H. Jick, "Relation of Childhood Gastrointestinal Disorders to Autism: Nested Case-Control Study Using Data from the UK General Practice Research Database," *BMJ* 325, no. 7361 (2002); W. Chen et al., "No Evidence for Links between Autism, MMR and Measles Virus," *Psychological Medicine* 34, no. 3 (2004); Loring Dales, Sandra Jo Hammer, and Natalie J. Smith, "Time Trends in Autism and in MMR Immunization Coverage in California," *JAMA* 285, no. 9 (2001); Robert L. Davis et al., "Measles-Mumps-Rubella and Other Measles-Containing Vaccines Do Not Increase the Risk for Inflammatory Bowel Disease: A Case-Control Study from the Vaccine Safety Datalink Project," *Archives of Pediatrics & Adolescent Medicine* 155, no. 3 (2001); Frank Destefano et al., "Age at First Measles-Mumps-Rubella Vaccination in Children with Autism and School-Matched Control Subjects: A Population-Based Study in Metropolitan Atlanta," *Pediatrics* 113, no. 2 (2004); A. Doja and W. Roberts, "Immunizations and Autism: A Review of the Literature," *Canadian Journal of Neurological Sciences* 33, no. 4 (2006); Yasmin D'Souza, Eric Fombonne, and Brian J. Ward, "No Evidence of Persisting Measles Virus in Peripheral Blood Mononuclear Cells from Children with Autism Spectrum Disorder.(Testing)," *Pediatrics* 118, no. 4 (2006); C. Paddy Farrington, Elizabeth Miller, and Brent Taylor, "MMR and Autism: Further Evidence against a Causal Association," *Vaccine* 19, no. 27 (2001); Eric Fombonne and Suniti Chakrabarti, "No Evidence for a New Variant of Measles-Mumps-Rubella-Induced Autism," *Pediatrics* 108, no. 4 (2001); Eric Fombonne et al., "Pervasive Developmental Disorders in Montreal, Quebec, Canada: Prevalence and Links with Immunizations," *Pediatrics* 118, no. 1 (2006); Hideo Honda, Yasuo Shimizu, and Michael Rutter, "No Effect of MMR Withdrawal on the Incidence of Autism: A Total Population Study," *Journal of Child Psychology and Psychiatry* 46, no. 6 (2005); Mady Hornig et al., "Lack of Association between Measles Virus Vaccine and Autism with Enteropathy: A Case-Control Study," *PLoS One* 3, no. 9 (2008); IOM, *Immunization Safety Review: Vaccines and Autism*, Vaccines and Autism (Washington, D.C.: National Academies Press, 2004); Anjali Jain et al., "Autism Occurrence by MMR Vaccine Status among US Children with Older Siblings with and without Autism," *JAMA* 313, no. 15 (2015); Ja Kaye, M. Del Mar Melero-Montes, and H. Jick, "Mumps, Measles, and Rubella Vaccine and the Incidence of Autism Recorded by General Practitioners: A Time Trend Analysis," *BMJ* 322, no. 7281 (2001); Kristin C. Klein and Emily B. Diehl, "Relationship between MMR Vaccine and Autism," *Annals of Pharmacotherapy* 38, no. 7–8 (2004); R. Lingam et al., "Prevalence of Autism and Parentally Reported Triggers in a North East London Population," *Archives of Disease in Childhood* 88, no. 8 (2003); Kreesten Meldgaard Madsen et al., "A Population-Based Study of Measles, Mumps, and Rubella Vaccination and Autism," *The New England Journal of Medicine* 347, no. 19 (2002); Annamari Makela, J. Nuorti, and Heikki Peltola, "Neurologic Disorders after Measles-Mumps-Rebella Vaccination," *Pediatrics* 110, no. 5 (2002); Dorota Mrożek-Budzyn, Agnieszka Kiełtyka, and Renata Majewska, "Lack of Association between Measles-Mumps-Rubella Vaccination and Autism in Children: A Case-Control Study," *The Pediatric Infectious Disease Journal* 29, no. 5 (2010); Heikki Peltola et al., "No Evidence for Measles, Mumps, and Rubella Vaccine-Associated Inflammatory Bowel Disease or Autism in a 14-Year Prospective Study," *Lancet* 351, no. 9112 (1998);

Jennifer Richler et al., "Is There a 'Regressive Phenotype' of Autism Spectrum Disorder Associated with the Measles-Mumps-Rubella Vaccine? A CPEA Study," *Journal of Autism and Developmental Disorders* 36, no. 3 (2006); Liam Smeeth et al., "MMR Vaccination and Pervasive Developmental Disorders: A Case-Control Study," *Lancet* 364, no. 9438 (2004); B. Taylor et al., "Autism and Measles, Mumps, and Rubella Vaccine: No Epidemiological Evidence for a Causal Association," *Lancet* 353, no. 9169 (1999); Brent Taylor et al., "Measles, Mumps, and Rubella Vaccination and Bowel Problems or Developmental Regression in Children with Autism: Population Study," *BMJ* 324, no. 7334 (2002); Tokio Uchiyama, Michiko Kurosawa, and Yutaka Inaba, "MMR-Vaccine and Regression in Autism Spectrum Disorders: Negative Results Presented from Japan," *Journal of Autism and Developmental Disorders* 37, no. 2 (2007).

81 Jennifer Keelan and Kumanan Wilson, "Balancing Vaccine Science and National Policy Objectives: Lessons from the National Vaccine Injury Compensation Program Omnibus Autism Proceedings," *American Journal of Public Health* 101, no. 11 (2011): 2016.

82 Ibid., 2018.

83 Zosia Kmietowicz, "Wakefield Is Struck Off for the 'Serious and Wide-Ranging Findings against Him'," *BMJ* 340 (2010): 1; T. S. Sathyanarayana Rao and Chittaranjan Andrade, "The MMR Vaccine and Autism: Sensation, Refutation, Retraction, and Fraud," *Indian Journal of Psychiatry* 53, no. 2 (2011).

84 Boaz Miller, "When Is Consensus Knowledge Based? Distinguishing Shared Knowledge from Mere Agreement," *An International Journal for Epistemology, Methodology and Philosophy of Science* 190, no. 7 (2013): 1294.

85 John Cook et al., "Quantifying the Consensus on Anthropogenic Global Warming in the Scientific Literature," *Environmental Research Letters* 8, no. 2 (2013); John Cook et al., "Consensus on Consensus: A Synthesis of Consensus Estimates on Human-Caused Global Warming," *Environmental Research Letters* 11, no. 4 (2016).

86 Diethelm and McKee, "Denialism: What Is It and How Should Scientists Respond?," 2.

87 Aechtner, "Distrust, Danger, and Confidence: A Content Analysis of the Australian Vaccination-Risks Network Blog," 25–26.

88 "Dr Gannon, AMA President, Declines Invitation to Answer Questions About Vaccination," AVN, https://avn.org.au/2017/10/dr-gannon-ama-president-declines-invitation-answer-questions-vaccination/.

89 "The Suffering Continues-Does the Government Care?," AVN, https://avn.org.au/2016/03/suffering-continues-government-care/.

90 Aechtner, *Media and the Science-Religion Conflict: Mass Persuasion in the Evolution Wars*, 67–68.

91 Richard E. Petty, John T. Cacioppo, and Rachel Goldman, "Personal Involvement as a Determinant of Argument-Based Persuasion," *Journal of Personality and Social Psychology* 41, no. 5 (1981); Richard E. Petty and John T. Cacioppo, *Communication and Persuasion: Central and Peripheral Routes to Attitude Change* (New York: Springer-Verlag, 1986), 142–43.

92 Elizabeth M. Perse, *Media Effects and Society* (Mahwah: Lawrence Erlbaum Associates, 2001), 89.

93 Petty and Cacioppo, *Communication and Persuasion*, 142–43.

94 Pamela M. Homer and Lynn R. Kahle, "Source Expertise, Time of Source Identification, and Involvement in Persuasion: An Elaborative Processing Perspective," *Journal of Advertising* 19, no. 1 (1990): 30–31; Joseph R. Priester and Richard E. Petty, "The Influence of Spokesperson Trustworthiness on

Message Elaboration, Attitude Strength, and Advertising Effectiveness," *Journal of Consumer Psychology* 13, no. 4 (2003); Zakary L. Tormala and Richard E. Petty, "Source Credibility and Attitude Certainty: A Metacognitive Analysis of Resistance to Persuasion," *Journal of Consumer Psychology* 14 (2004): 429; Uma R. Karmarkar and Zakary L. Tormala, "Believe Me, I Have No Idea What I'm Talking About: The Effects of Source Certainty on Consumer Involvement and Persuasion," *Journal of Consumer Research* 36, no. 6 (2010).

95   Michael E. Jones, "Celebrity Endorsements: A Case for Alarm and Concern for the Future," *New England Law Review* 15, no. 3 (1980).

96   Lisset Martinez-Berman, Lynn McCutcheon, and Ho P. Huynh, "Is the Worship of Celebrities Associated with Resistance to Vaccinations? Relationships between Celebrity Admiration, Anti-Vaccination Attitudes, and Beliefs in Conspiracy," *Psychology, Health & Medicine* 26, no. 9 (2021).

97   Aechtner, "Distrust, Danger, and Confidence: A Content Analysis of the Australian Vaccination-Risks Network Blog," 30; "Improving Evolution Advocacy: Translating Vaccine Interventions to the Evolution Wars."

98   Sarah Sorial, "The Legitimacy of Pseudo-Expert Discourse in the Public Sphere," *Metaphilosophy* 48, no. 3 (2017).

99   Aechtner, "Distrust, Danger, and Confidence: A Content Analysis of the Australian Vaccination-Risks Network Blog," 27–28; "Improving Evolution Advocacy: Translating Vaccine Interventions to the Evolution Wars," 30.

100   Hughes et al., "Development of a Codebook of Online Anti-Vaccination Rhetoric to Manage COVID-19 Vaccine Misinformation".

101   Tasha David, "Bad News on the Legal Challenge Front...but We Will Never Give up the Fight!," AVN, https://avn.org.au/2016/12/bad-news-legal-challenge-front-will-never-give-fight/.

102   Aechtner, *Media and the Science-Religion Conflict: Mass Persuasion in the Evolution Wars*, 180–83.

103   Petty and Cacioppo, *Communication and Persuasion*, 96–101.

104   Ibid., 212.

105   Janetta Lun et al., "(Why) Do I Think What You Think? Epistemic Social Tuning and Implicit Prejudice," *Journal of Personality and Social Psychology* 93, no. 6 (2007): 957.

106   Ibid., 958.

107   Gretchen B. Sechrist and Charles Stangor, "When Are Intergroup Attitudes Based on Perceived Consensus Information?: The Role of Group Familiarity," *Social Influence* 2, no. 3 (2007).

108   Perse, *Media Effects*, 115.

109   Danny Axsom, Shelly Chaiken, and Suzanne Yates, "Audience Response as a Heuristic Cue in Persuasion," *Journal of Personality and Social Psychology* 53, no. 1 (1987).

110   Daniel W. Fleitas, "Bandwagon and Underdog Effects in Minimal-Information Elections," *The American Political Science Review* 65, no. 2 (1971); Manfred Gartner, "Endogenous Bandwagon and Underdog Effects in a Rational Choice Model," *Public Choice* 25 (1976): 83.

111   Aechtner, "Distrust, Danger, and Confidence: A Content Analysis of the Australian Vaccination-Risks Network Blog," 27.

112   Dorey, "Nurses Don't Trust Vaccines".

113   Aechtner, *Media and the Science-Religion Conflict: Mass Persuasion in the Evolution Wars*, 178–80.

114   Robert Levine, *The Power of Persuasion: How We're Bought and Sold* (New Jersey: John Wiley & Sons, 2003), 33.

115 David M. Boush, Marian Friestad, and Peter Wright, *Deception in the Market-place: The Psychology of Deceptive Persuasion and Consumer Self Protection* (New York: Routledge, 2009), 70.

116 Richard F. Yalch and Rebecca Elmore-Yalch, "The Effect of Numbers on the Route to Persuasion," *Journal of Consumer Research* 11, no. 1 (1984): 526.

117 Aechtner, "Distrust, Danger, and Confidence: A Content Analysis of the Australian Vaccination-Risks Network Blog," 27.

118 Joel Cooper, Elizabeth A. Bennett, and Holly L. Sukel, "Complex Scientific Testimony: How Do Jurors Make Decisions?," *Law and Human Behavior* 20, no. 4 (1996); Carolyn L. Hafer, Kelly L. Reynolds, and Monika A. Obertynski, "Message Comprehensibility and Persuasion: Effects of Complex Language in Counterattitudinal Appeals to Laypeople," *Social Cognition* 14, no. 4 (1996).

119 Aechtner, "Distrust, Danger, and Confidence: A Content Analysis of the Australian Vaccination-Risks Network Blog."

4 Questioning safety
Danger and persuasion

There is a saying that has been informally attributed to Napoleon Bonaparte, which states that people "are moved by two levers only: fear and self-interest."[1] Even though this is a rather pessimistic saying, it is apparent that fear can truly be a powerful motivator. When it comes to vaccines, it is common for people to express fears over vaccine safety, including anxieties about potential adverse side effects and toxic ingredients (Chapter 2). Relatedly, one of the key elements of antivaccination media are messages about the dangers of getting vaccinated. These can include narratives about alleged vaccine injury, including claims that vaccines routinely cause autism and even death. Such stories not only feature apprehensions about vaccine components, but also anxieties about too many vaccines overloading immune systems. Similar alarming stories form the spine of counter-vaccine messages, and they have been a central feature of antivaccination claims since the 19th century. With these widespread ideas in mind, this chapter further considers the DCD of counter-vaccination messages by focusing on the Danger theme in antivaccine claims. This theme can include declarations that vaccines are risky because they are filled with toxic ingredients, or that vaccines routinely cause serious morbidities and mortality in recipients. While addressing such contentions, the chapter will examine how misperceptions of vaccine risks can directly impact vaccination uptake. Along the way it will expose eight of the most pervasive vaccination myths and their shortcomings, while introducing three persuasive cues that are frequently associated with the Danger theme.

Contemplating Danger

For the sake of simplicity, it is helpful to reduce people's attitudes towards possible vaccine risks into three basic options. The first of these involves a relative indifference to the prospect of vaccine dangers and the hypothetical risks of contracting a vaccine preventable disease. Instead, vaccines are assumed to be part of the accepted health routines of modern living, without much thought to danger or risks. The second option consists of risk perceptions primarily associated with the conceivable hazards of contracting

DOI: 10.4324/9781003312550-4

vaccine preventable diseases. Catching such an avoidable disease is understood to be risky enough to warrant getting vaccinated. The third option, on the other hand, involves assessing the possible dangers of vaccine-related side effects to be greater than those that result from contracting vaccine preventable illnesses.

Regarding the third option, in many countries numerous vaccine preventable diseases are relatively rare. People are often not exposed to the health repercussions caused by such illnesses as diphtheria, tetanus, or polio. For example, I grew up in Canada, where endemic polio had been eliminated through vaccination campaigns. In fact, one of the last outbreaks of wild poliomyelitis occurred in Canada the year before I was born, and as a result I did not witness the pathogen's effects until early adulthood. When I was 19 years old, I travelled overseas to West Africa, and it was only then that I met people with limb deformities caused by the disease. In West Africa I also witnessed a degree of public eagerness for vaccines that I had never encountered before. Fortunately, polio vaccines have significantly reduced global rates of polio. In 1988, over 125 countries struggled with endemic polio. By 2006, there were only 12 countries that still had active poliovirus transmission, which was an accomplishment achieved through vaccines.[2]

My own narrative reflects a common trend, whereby many people have never been exposed to the threat of vaccine preventable diseases. Consequently, without having directly witnessed the crippling morbidities caused by polio for themselves, the illness may not seem to be particularly worrisome. Out of sight, out of mind. As a result, for some, getting vaccinated

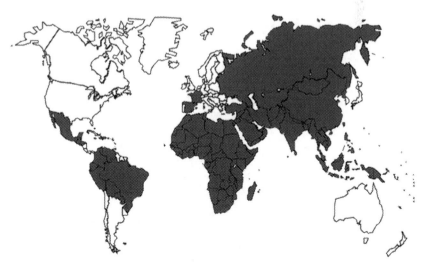

Figure 4.1 Countries with active polio transmission in 1988[3]

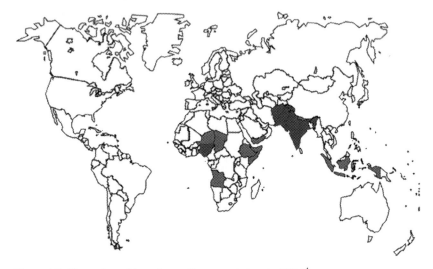

Figure 4.2 Countries with active polio transmission in 2006[4]

may appear to be more dangerous than polio itself. In that sense, when it comes to perceptions of danger, vaccines may be a victim of their own success.[5] If an individual has not witnessed the debilitative consequences of vaccine preventable diseases but has heard rumours about vaccine-related side effects, or even vaccine caused deaths, then the risk of getting vaccinated could be perceived to be much greater than catching the disease itself. As Canada's first chief health officer, Dr David Butler-Jones, stated regarding polio vaccination efforts:

> There's a Biblical story that says when the Israelites remembered God, they prospered. And when they prospered, they forgot God. That's a powerful allegory for our current efforts [in] polio eradication work. When we understand what succeeds and how it is we need to work together, we achieve. But, unfortunately, when we prosper, we often forget what got us there.[6]

In relation to this, research indicates that fears about vaccine side effects increase people's anxiety around vaccination.[7] This can cause people to believe that the danger of vaccinating against pathogens outweighs the risk of the diseases themselves. These risk calculations can be further skewed against getting vaccinated when populations have never been exposed to pathogens because they have been successfully controlled through vaccination.

Fears about vaccine side effects are also what make the Danger theme in antivaccination media so substantial because this motif taps into people's genuine fears. These are fears which are not counterbalanced by direct exposure to the potentially life-altering effects of vaccine preventable diseases like polio. What is also crucial about the power of fear messages is that when reports about vaccine risks are widely broadcasted by counter-vaccine groups, they can and have influenced real-world vaccine uptake. One study, for instance, analysed how vaccination rates dropped, and infections increased in countries where antivaccine groups spread stories about vaccine dangers.[8] The study examined how vaccine receipt changed from 1960 onwards when counter-vaccine movements began using mass media to circulate anecdotes about risks associated with diphtheria, tetanus, pertussis (DTP) combination vaccines in Sweden, Japan, Russia, and the United Kingdom. In these countries, well-organised antivaccination movements fought the use of these vaccines, which led to national immunisation programs being compromised. Each nation subsequently experienced increases in pertussis cases and significant outbreaks. In Sweden, DTP coverage decreased from 90% in 1974 to just 12% in 1979, and public fear toward the vaccine led the country to cease using it in 1979. As a result, Sweden would go on to report 10,000 cases per year. Japan experienced a pertussis epidemic in 1979 with more than 13,000 cases and 41 deaths reported. Russia and the UK also faced their own epidemics. Additionally, other countries, including Australia, Ireland, and Italy would go on to experience large outbreaks, which were also linked to antivaccine movements. As the authors of the study concluded, once "high vaccine uptake and herd immunity are attained, perceived vaccine risks tend to deter individuals from being vaccinated."[9]

Other research has identified how uptake rates of the measles, mumps, rubella (MMR) vaccine decreased after it was erroneously claimed that the vaccine caused autism (Chapter 3), and when the Prime Minister, Tony Blair, refused to state whether his son Leo had received the MMR vaccine.[10] This decline has been bound up with the spread of fear about the MMR vaccine by anti-immunisation lobby groups. Controversy and fear-inducing communications about MMR led to vaccine coverage falling from 92% to 80% at one time in England, with the rate dropping to as low as 58% in London.[11] Additionally, reports that the MMR vaccine is linked to cases of autism would go on to cultivate vaccine hesitancy for people around the world, and it is now hearsay that most people have heard before.

Along with MMR scare campaigns, a prominent case of stirred up fears impacting vaccination rates includes widespread stories about injury and death triggered by human papilloma virus (HPV) vaccines. Human papilloma viruses cause 70% of cervical cancers and pre-cancerous cervical lesions, yet today it is frightening stories about the apparent dangers of HPV vaccines that have become commonplace.[12] In 2009, a 14-year-old girl died 75 minutes after receiving an HPV vaccination in the United Kingdom. Though a public health official stated, "No link can be made between the death and the vaccine until all the facts are known and a post mortem takes place," the story would still go on to make headlines across the country. This involved the UK's news media actively spreading reports about the vaccine's possible risks, which helped fuel public fears about its safety.[13] In the end, the post mortem report of the 14-year-old girl who had died revealed that she had a "large malignant tumour in her chest, which caused her death."[14] This was a quintessential case of correlation not causation, but the spark of fear had already lit fires of anxiety (Chapter 1). Similar rumours of HPV-related injuries were then recounted elsewhere, including in a major Canadian newspaper, the *Toronto Star*, which featured a notorious article on HPV vaccines titled "A wonder drug's dark side." The *Star*, described as "Canada's highest-circulation newspaper," eventually acknowledged that its reporting was in error, clarifying that there "is no scientific medical evidence of any 'dark side' of this vaccine."[15] In fact, a large-scale study involving almost one million individuals found "no consistent evidence for a plausible association" between any serious disorders and the HPV vaccine.[16]

Nevertheless, as was the case in the UK, such reporting would stoke unfounded fears about the safety of HPV vaccines. Similar baseless but distressing claims were made by news outlets in Denmark and Ireland, which added to social media lobbying against HPV vaccines by concerned parents.[17] Such reports fuelled fears and led to declines in vaccine uptakes in both nations. Problematically, such stories about risk, and the anxiety that they induce, can be very difficult to displace once they have taken root in the imagination. This is why the influence of the Danger theme in antivaccination media should never be underestimated, even if all of the facts and all of the research declare that such fears are scientifically groundless.

Danger and the Arousal of Fear

The Danger theme and its influential might is, in part, linked with numerous vaccine myths and conspicuous persuasive cues that provoke fear. Counter-vaccine messages featuring this theme include personal accounts about the professed dangers of vaccines, including testimonies that vaccines can cause not only autism, but cerebral palsy and even schizophrenia.[18] Hence, antivaccination media frequently communicate that vaccines can cause such infirmities as "multiple sclerosis, brain inflammation, strokes, seizures, rheumatoid arthritis, disabling fatigue, cardiac arrhythmias, muscle pain and weakness, blood clots and death."[19] As noted above, such references to vaccine injury are also connected to alarming descriptions of vaccine ingredients. These ingredients include aluminium, along with other apparently dangerous "toxins" that should be feared due to their unknown health consequences.[20] These claims can be particularly effective when they are delivered alongside anecdotal personal stories about supposed vaccine-risks. For example, this might involve a mother telling audiences that vaccines injected into her children "caused them numerous health issues," and deprived them of "ever being able to live an independent life, of being able to fall in love or able to have a family of their own."[21] Stories like this can further insist that infant deaths result from vaccine-linked immune system overload, because as one antivaccination article claims, it is apparently "widely recognized that newborns have under-developed immune systems, which can be overwhelmed or shocked."[22] These sorts of stories are also not restricted to children, as counter-vaccine messages recurrently tell audiences of adult mortalities, indicating that, "More and more stories are emerging about babies, children and even adults dying within a short time after vaccination."[23]

Similar references to risk and danger can form the backbone of many antivaccination communications. The influence of these sorts of assertions is linked to the persuasive cue described as the *Arousal of Fear*. This cue is associated with threats of physical and emotional harm, which may be caused by an adversary or an opposing viewpoint. Researchers have found that the stimulation of emotions, and in particular fear, can kindle persuasion. In certain circumstances fear may cause audiences to rely upon other available peripheral cues within a message to make a decision.[24] If a message provokes strong sensations of fear, and then subsequently makes clear reassuring statements about the value of a solution to the fear-inducing problem, then message recipients seem to rely upon peripheral cues for persuasion rather than engaging in more mentally taxing central route processing. For instance, if a communication stimulates fear in an audience about vaccines, and then clearly proposes a seemingly effective answer to the problem, audiences may simply rely on the communicator's perceived credibility when choosing to accept this recommended answer. However, if a clear reassuring solution to the fear-engendering message is not provided then fear itself serves as a sort of cue to induce central route message processing.

Such appeals are also of note regarding vaccine hesitancy because arousing fear and evoking feelings of anxiety have been found to increase tendencies to share fear-stimulating messages with others.[25] That is to say, people are more likely to pass on information and stories, perhaps about vaccines, that they find worrying. Furthermore, in view of the Cultural Cognition Thesis, people seem inclined to experience negative emotions such as fear when risks are perceived to threaten to their own cultural values. If a potential risk is deemed to be a threat to the values held closely by an individual, then a fear response will be consistent with the perceived threat itself.[26] With that in mind, if mandatory vaccination policies are thought to overstep someone's closely held cultural values about people's individual rights to make medical choices for their families without government interference, then an individual may experience feelings of alarm in response to such compulsory legislation.

Research has found that hearing anecdotal stories about vaccine injuries can influence vaccine decision-making.[27] This is because fear-inducing stories can increase the perceived risk of vaccine side effects. In fact, it seems that people are more likely to perceive vaccines to be risky if they have encountered a greater number of online anecdotal stories about vaccine side effects.[28] Broadly speaking, anecdotal stories have been found to impact audiences, and are also often favoured to over non-narrative, factual information.[29] We prefer to hear and internalise a good story over statistics and fact claims. As a one report has noted about the power of stories and people's assessment of medical risks, "A good narrative trumps facts," and a narrative with an alarming, fear-kindling personal story about vaccine injury can be particularly influential.[30]

The Contrast Principle and Negativity Effect

Intriguingly, the anecdotal stories about vaccine injuries tied to the Danger theme often incorporate noticeable comparisons. These comparisons can include frightening narratives that contrast an individual's health before and after receiving vaccinations. Such narratives emphasise the disparities between the reported pre-vaccine health and post-vaccine injuries or even death in both children and adults.[31] Also, the apparent knowledge and truthfulness of vaccine-sceptics are compared with the lack of knowledge and dishonesty maintained by vaccination supporters. This includes comparing the "multiple falsehoods" of pro-vaccine advocates with "genuine" scientific facts that are claimed to back up vaccine-scepticism.[32] Antivaccinationists are described as sincerely seeking to inform the public without corporate invested interests, using "unbiased" facts about vaccine risks. These accounts are contrasted with caricatures of their opponents, who are said to employ "the most cynical form of deceit to appeal to parents' hard-wired biological instincts to protect their babies from harm by selling them a 'magic forcefield.'"[33] Comparisons are also expressed in posts that contrast the pro-vaccination news media's apparent lack of research, fraudulent "hate speech" and parroting of "pharmaceutical propaganda," with what is described as legitimate, scientific vaccine data emphasized by truth-seeking antivaccinationists.[34] Such comparisons relate to the persuasive cue described as the *Contrast Principle and Negativity Effect*. This persuasive technique is central to comparative advertising, and it involves weighing up a marketed product or rival idea against the competition's merchandise or viewpoint to highlight that the former is a superior option.[35]

Comparative advertising has remained a common marketing strategy. A well-known example of it includes the Apple Inc.'s *Get a Mac* advertising campaign, which showcased two actors personifying rival Mac and PC computers.[36] These commercials were explicitly designed to be comparative, and they used the two actors to emphasise the advantages of Macintosh computers while accenting the apparent drawbacks of PC hardware and software.[37] In various research conditions, this tactic has been said to make ads far more effective than non-comparative promotions at garnering audience attention and alertness, while heightening message recall, increasing purchase intentions, and cultivating buying behaviours.[38] Comparative advertising has been found to be most effective in the USA, with varying persuasion effects recorded across different cultural contexts; though the approach has generated convincing results in other parts of the world.[39]

The rationale underlying this practice is the *Contrast Principle*, which suggests that when two items or ideas are presented side-by-side, the differences between the two are accentuated for persuasion purposes. With respect to such contrast influences, Cialdini has explained that when we "lift a light object first and then lift a heavy object, we will estimate the second object to be heavier than if we had lifted it without first lifting the light one."[40] This same psychological tendency can be used to sway audiences towards a product or concept more successfully than if no comparison had been made at all. Such contrast is not only persuasive, but it has also been described as "virtually undetectable."[41] Consequently, contrast effects can markedly colour choices and influence persuasion when there is low-to-mid message elaboration likelihood.[42] Contrast may be unfairly structured to favour a particular product or concept, and include ridicule and biased caricatures of a competitor.[43] For this reason, direct comparative advertising has sometimes been banned and is often legally regulated.[44]

Notably, contrast that is antagonistic towards an opponent, which emphasises the negative attributes of a competitor's ideas or products is associated with what has been described as the *Negativity Effect*. With regard to comparative advertising, studies indicate that comparisons which denigrate a rival product tend to be more effective.[45] Associatively, it has been demonstrated that "negative information is often more powerful in creating attitudes (i.e., it is weighted more heavily) than is positive information of equal extremity."[46] As a consequence, negative messages in opposition to a particular product or idea have stronger, relatively automatic persuasion effects in comparison to positive information that supports goods or concepts. In political election campaigns, for instance, negative information and opinions regarding what voters disagree with prove to be more influential than positive information in agreement with what the electorate supports. In the end, attitudes that are expressed as being *against* something prove to be more resilient than those that are *for* a position. In this way negative information that deliberately opposes an idea acts as a type of peripheral cue towards the contrary position.[47] Altogether, the Contrast Principle and the Negativity Effect are frequently in play throughout counter-vaccine danger narratives, including the persistent myth that vaccines of all sorts cause autism. A related question includes, where did this myth come from in the first place and what is story behind it?

Myth #6: Vaccines cause autism

One of the most enduring fears about vaccines, which remains a major component of the Danger theme in antivaccination media, is that vaccination increases the risk of autism spectrum disorder (ASD) in children.[48] ASD is described by the Centers for Disease Control and Prevention as a "developmental disability that can cause significant social, communication, and behavioral challenges."[49] The CDC has further explained:

> People with ASD often have problems with social, emotional, and communication skills. They might repeat certain behaviors and might not want change in their daily activities. Many people with ASD also have different ways of learning, paying attention, or reacting to things. Signs of ASD begin during early childhood and typically last throughout a person's life.[50]

Though researchers have gained important knowledge about autism over recent years, scientists still are not absolutely certain of its causes. Nevertheless, despite uncertainties, there has been no association found between vaccines and ASD.

As recounted in Chapter 3, fears that vaccines cause autism were triggered when the British surgeon, Andrew Wakefield, co-published an article that raised the possibility of a link between the measles, mumps, rubella vaccine, chronic inflammation of the digestive tract, and autism in children.[51] Even though the study maintained that the authors had not found a causative link between the vaccine and autism, Wakefield stoked public anxieties by making public announcements warning that the MMR vaccine should be suspended until further safety analyses could be completed.[52] In the end, the academic study that asserted that an autism–MMR link exists was found to be based on serious scientific misconduct.[53] Still, the claim that MMR increased vaccine risks sparked a substantial number of academic studies, which have all found no link between autism and vaccination.[54] Instead, research indicates that there are likely several potential causes of ASD. There seems to be a link between genetic variables and risk of autism, while children born to older parents are more at risk of developing ASD.[55] There also appear to be prenatal and neonatal risk factors associated with autism, which occur before children receive vaccinations.[56] Autism seems to arise during the development of the foetus' nervous system while it is still in the womb.

The connection between ASD diagnoses and vaccines is also likely to be influenced by correlational observations. Many symptoms of autism are detected around the same time that children receive vaccines, such as MMR, so a causal linkage is perceived even though the circumstances are coincidental. Additionally, diagnoses of autism have increased over past decades, leading people to question whether vaccines are the cause of this uptick in numbers.[57] However, increased ASD diagnoses are likely due to changes in medical criteria used to determine what is included within the spectrum, as well as greater awareness of ASD maintained by practitioners who are able to diagnose symptoms. In the end, there is no scientific evidence connecting vaccines with autism, yet the vaccine–autism myth persists. It remains one of the most serious falsehoods of the Danger theme in antivaccination media, and it is a myth that policymakers and medical professionals need to keep in mind, despite being scientifically discredited.[58] In addition to Wakefield's debacle of refuted MMR–autism claims, vaccines have also been accused of leading to numerous other health concerns. One of the most prominent of such allegations includes assertions that vaccines are tied to allergic diseases and stressing that vaccines can routinely cause severe allergic reactions.

Myth #7: Vaccines and allergies

Allergies have become more prevalent in developed regions of the world throughout the late 20th century.[59] A leading theory to explain this increase is the *hygiene hypothesis*, which suggests that improved hygiene leads to a "decreasing incidence of infections in western countries and more recently in developing countries."[60] It is thought that this decline correlates with a rise in allergic diseases. The assumption is that exposure to microbes and infections during childhood contributes to the health of the immune system, which subsequently protects against allergic diseases. Improved sanitation, hygienic practices, and other lifestyle changes occurring in developed countries, therefore, limit such pathogen exposure and results are increased allergy rates, but this does not occur when children experience more infections. For example, it has been found that even living "in a large family, attending day care early in life, and growing up on a farm" amplify exposure to infections, and this has been "shown to reduce the risk of asthma and allergies."[61] Similarly, being "exposed to food-borne and oro-fecal infections at early age" has been linked with "a decreased prevalence of hay fever and asthma."[62] As Thomas Platts-Mills concluded, increases in allergies "did not start until the most important changes in hygiene had been achieved."[63] Furthermore, "In keeping with this, the forms of allergic disease that are most common in developed countries are not present" in other less developed nations, such as "Kenyan, Ethiopian, and Ecuadorian villages or in poor areas of a major city in Ghana."[64]

The hygiene hypothesis has gone on to face scientific criticism. This is because researchers have pointed out that several complex factors may be leading to increased allergic diseases, and these influences are not necessarily associated with hygiene changes.[65] In light of such increases in allergic diseases in various parts of the world, it has also been claimed that vaccines are to blame for this phenomenon. Counter-vaccine leaders profess it is no accident that upsurges in allergic diseases and other ailments have "coincided with a sudden increase in the number and doses of vaccines on the schedules in those countries."[66] This includes claims that vaccine ingredients are directly responsible for "causing allergies" in people. Vaccines, it is alleged, can "easily set up subsequent allergy to any protein in the injection," which can generate allergies "to common foods such as eggs, milk, peanuts, tree nuts and grains."[67] Consequently, some antivaccination messages assert that not vaccinating is actually a positive lifestyle choice, which helps to build "protection against asthma, allergies."[68] Additionally, the Danger theme of antivaccination media also includes emphasising that serious risks associated with vaccinating include experiencing severe allergic reactions. Broadly speaking then, antivaccine media can link allergies to vaccination in one way or another, so it is essential to investigate the evidence around such claims.

Unmistakably, there has been an escalation of allergic diseases in developed nations, and it is also true that people receive more vaccines today than they have in the past. It might be tempting, therefore, to connect these two trends. With that possibility in mind, researchers have investigated whether vaccination can be associated with allergies. Importantly, a significant study that analysed available research data concluded that vaccines "do not increase the risk of developing allergic disease."[69] Research has repeatedly failed to confirm findings that childhood vaccinations are responsible for the increased prevalence of allergic illnesses in developed countries.[70] Whereas claims that vaccines, as well as antibiotics, might be leading to allergies are "not founded on scientific evidence," a number of key reports "have in fact shown that all types of vaccination strategies do not result in either increased or decreased risk of asthma and allergies up to school age."[71] It should also be noted that even if a link between allergies and vaccination is eventually uncovered, this would not necessarily denote that vaccinations are unbeneficial. The overall benefits of reducing infections from potentially life altering or deadly diseases arguably outweigh possible increases in allergies.

It is also the case that severe allergic reaction resulting from vaccines are extremely rare. These incidents can occur if an individual is allergic to specific vaccine ingredients, including egg proteins that may be present in an influenza vaccine, or gelatin in live attenuated vaccines, as well as antibiotics in inactivated poliovirus vaccines. It has been reported that anaphylaxis, which is a serious allergic reaction, occurs in approximately 0.0002% of cases of the measles vaccine and the Hepatitis B vaccine.[72] An Australian study found that anaphylaxis occurred in approximately 0.0026% of HPV doses, while such reactions were observed in only 0.0001% of doses of the Men-C, conjugated meningococcal C, vaccine.[73] By comparison, a mathematician has estimated that the chance of being struck by lightning in Australia is 0.008%.[74] This puts matters into perspective because it means that there is a significantly greater likelihood of being struck by lightning, a very rare occurrence, than of experiencing a severe allergic reaction to a vaccine.

Severe allergic reactions to vaccines are astoundingly uncommon. It should also be remembered that such outcomes occur due to pre-existent allergies to certain ingredients, and not because vaccines are themselves causing new forms of allergic disease not already present before vaccine receipt. Additionally, the incredibly unlikely possibility of experiencing a severe allergic reaction is eclipsed by the much more probable chance of suffering a life-altering illness, or even death, from numerous vaccine preventable diseases.

Myth #8: Vaccines cause autoimmune diseases

Much like allergies, it has also been recognised that autoimmune diseases have been increasing in developed regions of the world. In fact, auto-immune diseases affect approximately 5% of people in developed countries.[75] As with allergies, this trend has been associated with hygiene hypothesis factors.[76] In response to such observations, antivaccination media have also connected this development to vaccines. For instance, a 2019 antivaccination article asked audiences, "Is it not feasible that our modern lifestyle incorporating cradle-to-grave vaccination has created a huge population of autoimmune and immune-compromised people?"[77] Another post claimed that in some cases HPV vaccines can make the "occurrence of autoimmune reactions across the body almost unavoidable."[78] Similar assertions mark the Danger theme in antivaccination messages, which together communicate that a common risk of vaccines is the weakening of the immune system and autoimmune disorders.

As it turns out, antivaccinationists are not the only people to suggest that vaccines may be leading to autoimmune diseases. Nevertheless, more "rigorous investigation has failed to confirm most of the allegations."[79] There are, however, two types of rare conditions that have been linked to vaccine receipt. One of these includes the risk of developing *Guillain-Barré Syndrome*, a rare but serious disorder that involves the immune system attacking the peripheral nervous system, leading to muscle weakness and paralysis. Approximately 70% of those afflicted with the syndrome recover fully, though possible long-term problems can include being unable to walk without assistance, weakness to muscles and ongoing tiredness.[80] Though the causes of the syndrome are not fully understood, it often occurs following a viral or bacterial infection. In 1976, there was an increased risk of acquiring Guillain-Barré Syndrome detected from the swine flu vaccine.[81] Increased risk of the syndrome has also been associated with the Influenza A, H1N1 vaccine, which was reported to be "about 1.6 excess cases per million people vaccinated."[82] This equates to approximately a 0.00016% increase in Guillain-Barré Syndrome amongst the population. Importantly, this risk is "judged substantially lower than the risk for severe influenza and influenza-related complications."[83] Other studies have also reported finding no significant link between Guillain-Barré Syndrome and other influenza vaccines, while instead there was a strong association between the syndrome and natural flu infection.[84] Consequently, there is a far greater risk of acquiring Guillain-Barré Syndrome from natural influenza infections than from a vaccine.

A second autoimmune risk that has been associated with vaccination is the development of a rare condition known as *idiopathic thrombocytopenic purpura* (ITP), also referred to as *immune thrombocytopenia*, following the measles, mumps, rubella vaccine and influenza vaccines. ITP also gained significant public attention when it was said to arise from COVID-19 vaccines.[85] Idiopathic thrombocytopenic purpura is a rare disorder that can sometimes follow viral infections. It results in a decrease in the number of platelets in the blood, causing blood to stop clotting normally.[86] This can lead to bruising, blood in stool and urine, nosebleeds, and bleeding from the gums. In the majority of cases ITP is not serious, and it often resolves within six months in children. It has been reported that the disorder can occur in approximately 1 in every 30,000 children who are vaccinated with MMR, where it was also found that "MMR-associated ITP is rare, self-limited, and non-life threatening."[87] However, as researchers have explained, it is "noteworthy that the risk of thrombocytopenia after natural rubella (one in 3,000) or measles (one in 6,000) infections is much greater than after vaccination."[88] Likewise, both COVID-19 and influenza infections have been associated with ITP complications.[89] Also, as with MMR vaccines, the risk of ITP events occurring as a result of natural COVID-19 or influenza infections is also substantially higher and prolonged than from vaccines.[90]

A key takeaway is that the risks associated with acquiring ITP from natural infections is pointedly greater than dangers connected with influenza, MMR or COVID-19 vaccines, while not vaccinating can also include hazards accompanying natural infection. Therefore, if people are fearful of idiopathic thrombocytopenic purpura, the risks of experiencing ITP complications are actually far greater in naturally acquired influenza, measles, rubella, or SARS-CoV-2 infection, than they are with vaccines. Somewhat analogously, the similar conclusions have been made regarding COVID-19 vaccines and myocarditis. A rare risk of contracting myocarditis, inflammation of a heart muscle, after receiving SARS-CoV-2 mRNA vaccines made pandemic headlines alongside ITP fears.[91] However, researchers found that myocarditis and long-term heart problems are associated with COVID-19 infection itself.[92] Additionally, the chances of experiencing heart inflammation from SARS-CoV-2 itself are substantially higher than they are following vaccination. Once again, while vaccines are not without risk, the probability of developing autoimmune disorders or myocarditis following vaccination is much less likely than what occurs when people are infected with vaccine-preventable diseases.

Myth #9: Vaccines cause the diseases that they are designed to prevent

In addition to worries about allergies and autoimmune diseases, another common fear is that vaccines cause the diseases that they are meant to avert. This idea has been widely spread about SARS-CoV-2 vaccines. For example, it was embodied in a placard displayed at a Canadian protest against Bill Gates that exclaimed "THE VAX GIVES YOU COVID."[93] It was also put into words on a sign posted by an Australian organic food shop that rejected COVID-19 safety measures. The sign stated, "to protect our customers and each other, if you have had any vaccine in the last 10 to 14 days please do not enter."[94] Regarding such fears, vaccines can sometimes cause mild symptoms, including drowsiness, fever, nausea, and swelling at the injection site. Remember that vaccines harness our immune systems by training the body to recognise and combat pathogens. This training occurs when the immune system reacts to vaccine ingredients, and it may involve experiencing symptoms that resemble an actual infection. Such symptoms can indicate that your body is undergoing the necessary immunological responses required to ensure future immunity.

However, the vast majority of vaccines simply cannot cause the diseases that they are designed to prevent. This is because most vaccines contain only an antigen component of a pathogen, rather than a whole weakened or killed pathogen (Chapter 1). For instance, subunit and toxoid vaccines are based upon antigen constituents, while killed/inactivated vaccines contain the dead remains of pathogens, which cannot replicate and cause disease. mRNA vaccines contain a sequence of viral messenger ribonucleic acid, which codes for only one fragment of a virus's proteins that is merely a part of a pathogen that cannot replicate and cause disease. The question then remains, what about live attenuated vaccines?

When individuals are infected with communicable diseases, a pathogen can be spread from person to person through coughing, sneezing, direct bodily contact, or through ingestion. During an infection, a pathogen replicates in the body and is subsequently released into the environment where it can infect others. This is referred to as bacterial or viral *shedding*. A concern is whether live attenuated vaccines can also lead to disease and shedding associated with natural infections. Importantly, live attenuated vaccines generally do not cause disease in people who have healthy immune systems, because the weakened pathogen is not able to replicate fast enough. The same is also true for most people who do not have healthy immune systems, but people with immunodeficiency disorders are generally not given live attenuated vaccines.[95]

Nevertheless, in some incredibly rare cases live attenuated vaccines *can* cause viral shedding. It has been observed that the rotavirus vaccine can cause shedding in stool, while the rubella component of the MMR vaccine can shed into breastmilk.[96] The varicella vaccine can also lead to the spreading of chickenpox if a vaccine recipient develops a rash following vaccination. However, the chances of this occurring are minute. As the CDC has reported, "Worldwide, since 1995, only 11 healthy vaccinated people have been documented as spreading [varicella] vaccine virus to 13 unvaccinated persons."[97] Such cases are exceedingly uncommon because, even if the live attenuated vaccine virus is shed, in its weakened state it replicates far less frequently than naturally occurring pathogens. This means that less virus can be shed to infect others. Additionally, even if vaccine viral shedding occurs, it is unlikely to make other people sick because the pathogen's weakened state is designed to elicit an immune response without causing significant disease symptoms. For these reasons, shed vaccine viruses rarely cause illnesses in others, and are highly unlikely to lead to outbreaks.

The oral polio vaccine (OPV) is one of the few vaccines that has been shown to cause disease. This vaccine was introduced in the late 1950s, and it is no longer employed in many parts of the world.[98] Countries such as the USA, UK, Canada, and Australia have opted to use a killed/inactivated polio vaccine instead. This inactivated vaccine contains no live virus, and it has proven to be one of the safest vaccines available.[99] Unfortunately, the inactivated poliovirus vaccine costs approximately five times that of the OPV, and it also requires sterile syringes.[100] As a result, some regions have continued to use the oral polio vaccine. Importantly, the OPV can lead to viral shedding significant enough to spread to others, though cases of this happening are exceedingly rare.[101] For instance, the World Health Organization has indicated, "Since 2000, more than 10 billion doses of OPV have been administered to nearly 3 billion children worldwide."[102] Yet during this time there were only 760 vaccine-derived poliovirus cases. This is of particular concern for people living in under-vaccinated areas. As the WHO has maintained, in such instances the problem is effectively "not with the vaccine itself, but low vaccination coverage," because only in low vaccinated communities can the vaccine-linked poliovirus spread.[103]

In the final analysis then, most vaccines cannot lead to disease, because they only contain antigen parts, inactivated pathogens, or limited mRNA code. There are, however, very rare cases where live attenuated vaccines may result in shedding, though this is unlikely to cause infection and illness in others. With this in mind, it is important to consider the odds of pathogen shedding arising from vaccines in contrast with natural infections. When someone receives the varicella vaccine, for example, the likelihood of that individual spreading the attenuated chickenpox virus is highly improbable. Yet people who are naturally infected with chickenpox will most certainly shed the highly contagious virus. This naturally occurring virus can lead to such complications as pneumonia, secondary bacterial infections, foetal malformations when pregnant mothers are infected, and even death in immunosuppressed individuals.[104] When it comes to health safety and viral shedding, therefore, the safety odds significantly favour the varicella vaccination, as well as other live attenuated vaccines.

Myth #10: Vaccines contain dangerous toxins

Perhaps the most widely circulated legend about vaccination dangers, that is often connected in one way or another to the previous myths discussed in this chapter, relates to allegations about the noxious ingredients contained in vaccines. Arguably, the most intimidating aspects of vaccination include the possibility of experiencing pain and discomfort from a needle, as well as worries about having unknown substances injected into us. For many people, the prospect of having such ingredients as aluminium, formaldehyde, mercury, and potential toxins introduced into a child's body through vaccination may sound especially frightening. Taking such fears into account, it is revealing that antivaccination messages frequently insist that vaccines contain hazardous chemicals, which are said to be present in quantities large enough to lead to serious health problems.[105] Overall, the repeated claim is that "vaccines are toxic and poisonous and made from undesirable, bizarre products."[106] These types of claims ought to be taken seriously, because fears about vaccine ingredients may be leading to undue vaccine hesitancy.

It is true that aluminium, formaldehyde, and mercury can be toxic to humans. Such chemicals are also included in certain vaccine ingredients as adjuvants and expedients. Nonetheless, even though it may seem counter-intuitive, these two realities do not indicate that vaccines are toxic or dangerous. This is because vaccines contain these ingredients in only miniscule amounts, where such substances are not harmful in small quantities. Also, despite having frightening names, such chemicals are frequently found naturally in our own bodies, while others are contained in healthy foods that people consume on a regular basis. Formaldehyde, for example, is included in some vaccines to inactivate viruses, or to detoxify bacterial toxins. Yet formaldehyde also occurs in the environment, and it is produced in the body as part of normal metabolic functions. In fact, "Studies have shown that for a newborn of average weight of 6–8 pounds, the amount of formaldehyde in their body is 50–70 times higher than the upper amount that they could receive from a single dose of a vaccine or from vaccines administered over time."[107]

Another ingredient that causes anxieties, and which is featured throughout counter-vaccine messages, is mercury. This chemical element is found in the vaccine preservative thimerosal that is used in some multi-dose flu vaccines. Worries were raised that this mercury-containing preservative was causing autism in children. Like formaldehyde, mercury is also naturally occurring, but when it exists in the form methylmercury it can be toxic to people. However, thimerosal contains mercury in the form of ethylmercury, which is processed differently in the body, and is rapidly eliminated from our systems.[109] All the same, thimerosal was removed from many vaccines due to persistent fears. Its use was discontinued as a precaution stemming from public anxiety, not because it was toxic. Numerous studies then analysed rates of autism in countries such as Sweden and Denmark, where the use of thimerosal in vaccines had been halted. These analyses found that diagnoses of autism actually increased in the years following the elimination of thimerosal.[110] Thimerosal simply could not have been the cause of autism, because rates of autism diagnoses trended upward when no thimerosal vaccines were in use.

Researchers also sought to measure whether there was any impact of different quantities of thimerosal in vaccines on autism, childhood development and early motor skills, but no study has found any evidence of negative effects.[111] There has been no consistent link uncovered between thimerosal use or disuse and autism. As Michael Shevell and Eric Fombonne

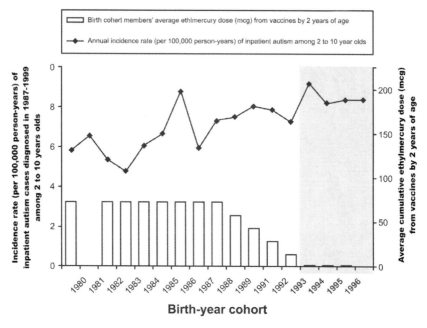

Figure 4.3 Incidence rate of autism in children contrasted with ethylmercury dose from vaccines in Sweden (data unavailable for 1981)[108]

have concluded, the belief that "excessive thimerosal exposure may be causally linked to the occurrence of an autistic spectrum disorder has many of the features of an urban legend," rather than any basis in scientific evidence.[112] Consequently, even though some vaccines can contain formaldehyde, aluminium, and mercury-containing thimerosal, it is important to remember that such substances are often naturally occurring, and we can regularly consume these same chemicals in normal diets. Also, trace amounts of these ingredients in vaccines are miniscule, while no links have been found between thimerosal and autism or other negative outcomes. Yet, despite the preponderance of evidence, counter-vaccine media has been outspoken in asking questions about vaccine ingredients, implying that there are vaccination–autism links. This trend is connected to the persuasive cue described as *Asking Questions*.

Asking Questions and the Danger theme

The very first blog post of an antivaccination lobby group that I have studied begins with the following remark: "Our children. Is there anything we wouldn't do for them?"[113] This simple rhetorical question characterises a major topic in counter-vaccine media, which involves emphasising that one of the community's primary goals is to keep children safe and to protect parents' autonomy of healthcare choices. At the same time, it also points to how rhetorical questions are sometimes used in antivaccine media, and the conceivable persuasiveness of such inquiries.[114]

Asking Questions can be identified as the use of rhetorical queries, also known as *eroteme*, which involves asking a question without expecting an answer because the answer itself is strongly implied within the question itself. The rhetorical devices termed *hypophora* and *anacoenosis* can also be integrated into this persuasive cue.[115] Hypophora comprises asking a question and then immediately answering it, while anacoenosis involves asking the opinion of an audience in a way that implies common interest without needing an answer.[116] The following account from the advertising veteran, J. Scott Armstrong, encapsulates how this message variable can operate. "I was sitting in a lecture and struggling to stay awake," notes Armstrong.[117] "Then the lecturer asked a question. It jolted me awake. The lecturer then went on to answer his own question." As this succinct narrative illustrates, rhetorical questions have been found to enhance message processing in audiences, especially in cases where individuals initially exhibit little interest in a communication's claims.[118] Consequently, asking these sorts of rhetorical questions can be used as a type of persuasive cue to stimulate thinking about message content in low elaboration likelihood contexts.[119]

These different varieties of questions are used throughout antivaccination messages to sow doubt about the expertise of doctors.[120] Other questions raise uncertainties about the safety of vaccine ingredients, while audiences are also asked whether scientific data truly supports the safety and effectiveness of vaccines.[121] Similarly, antivaccine media ask questions about the moral character and motives of pro-vaccination advocates.[122] In the end, cases of eroteme, hypophora, and anacoenosis occur alongside other major antivaccination claims. This includes reinforcing the message that vaccine-sceptics resist vaccines because they want to protect and care for their children. As one antivaccinationist concluded with hypophora: "You want to know the most important reason why I and many other parents don't vaccinate their child? We do it because we love them and want to protect them, just like you love your child and no amount of legislation or shaming tactics will ever change that."[123] It also involves asking tenaciously whether vaccines overload children's immune systems.

Myth #11: Vaccines can cause immune system overload

One of the leading concerns expressed about vaccines is that they may overload a child's immune system, resulting in detrimental effects.[124] It is commonly thought that an infant's immune system is too immature to receive numerous vaccinations, and therefore, multiple vaccines, delivered too soon in a child's life, will overload its body.[125] This idea has led to claims that vaccine-caused overloads result in any number of adverse reactions, including weakened immune systems, autism, as well as other chronic ailments and even death. As one antivaccination article has declared, infant deaths can result from vaccine-linked immune system overload, because it "is widely recognized that newborns have under-developed immune systems, which can be overwhelmed or shocked."[126] These concerns have been cited as leading to approximately 10–15% of parents delaying vaccination or using alternative vaccine schedules to those recommended by experts.[127]

At first glance, this might all appear to be intuitive. Human babies are born without the ability to hold up their own heads. Newborns are unable to walk, and they appear to be underdeveloped compared to many other animals at birth, such as precocial species like horses that can often begin walking within minutes of being born. Consequently, if a human's musculoskeletal system is not fully developed for walking at birth, does it not also make sense that a baby's immune system is unprepared for vaccines? Unfortunately, while this judgement seems to make sense, it is incorrect. A newborn's immune system is equipped to protect the body from infection at birth. In fact, babies are exposed to pathogens within minutes of being born, and children's immune systems are continually fighting off bacteria and viruses. A child's body actually deals with a far greater number of pathogens on a day-to-day basis than they are exposed to in vaccine doses.[128] As the authors of one study concluded, "we would predict that if 11 vaccines were given to infants at one time, then about 0.1% of the immune system would be 'used up.'"[129] As a matter of fact, because the immune system is constantly replenishing white blood cells, a "vaccine never really 'uses up' a fraction of the immune system" at all.[130] Vaccines do not overload infants' bodies, because the immune system is fit for purpose to handle far more pathogens, on a regular basis, than are contained in multiple vaccines.

Research dedicated to studying the claim that too many vaccines, too soon, is hazardous has resulted in no evidence to suggest that receiving multiple shots overburdens a child's immune system.[131] When children who received all their vaccines on-time in the first seven months of their lives were compared with children who had delayed vaccines, or received no vaccines at all, there were no differences found in 42 neuropsychological health outcomes.[132] Instead, while receiving all vaccines does not overload the immune system, and does not result in negative health outcomes, under-vaccinating children predictably puts children at risk of vaccine preventable diseases.[133] Furthermore, research has indicated that when children receive multiple vaccines, they do not experience weakened immune systems. Alternatively, vaccinated children demonstrated fewer illnesses than did unvaccinated kids, suggesting that vaccinated individuals might boast more robust immune responses. As researchers in Germany concluded: "Our study revealed that children who received vaccination against diphtheria, pertussis, tetanus, Hib and poliomyelitis simultaneously within the third month of life do not exhibit enhanced frequencies of infectious disease-associated symptoms."[134] In fact, the "frequencies of infection-associated symptoms were found to be significantly reduced." Additionally, in one study researchers examined whether they could identify any association between autism and receiving the full complement of vaccines at an early age. They found no such connection and stated that their "results indicate that parental concerns that their children are receiving too many vaccines in the first 2 years of life or too many vaccines at a single doctor visit are not supported in terms of an increased risk of autism."[135]

It is indisputable that academic studies refute the commonly held belief that too many vaccines, administered too soon in a child's life overload or weaken the immune system. There is also no factual basis to claims that receiving multiple vaccines leads to autism or other health concerns. By contrast, it seems that vaccinated children potentially exhibit fewer infectious-disease symptoms overall, while not immunising exposes infants to the risk of catching a vaccine preventable illness. What this also points to are the ways in which our health intuitions can be erroneous, even if they seem to be common-sensical at first glance. Infants are physically vulnerable and unable to fend for themselves. Consequently, it could be reasonable to assume that their immune systems are also underdeveloped and at risk of overloading from multiple vaccines. Though that assumption might *feel* logical, it turns out to be well off target from medical findings. Similar health intuitions may also lie behind the pervasive myth that vaccines are unsafe during pregnancy. Where infants are perceived to be at risk, pregnant women and their unborn children too are mistakenly thought to be in greater danger from vaccines.

Myth #12: Vaccines are unsafe during pregnancy

Debates about vaccine safety during pregnancy can be a significant online topic.[136] Questions about pregnancy and vaccine safety were also hastened by the COVID-19 pandemic, during which pregnant women across the world exhibited much lower vaccination rates than the rest of the public.[137] In the midst of such controversies, counter-vaccine messages vented distrust regarding scientific safety data and the effectiveness of vaccines, as well as mistrust of health authorities and vaccine producers. This includes conveying fears that vaccination might cause pregnant mothers and their unborn children harm, with the implication that "vaccines in pregnancy are not 'entirely safe.'"[138] Such claims are especially concerning because it has long been observed that pregnant women and their children actually face elevated risks from vaccine preventable diseases.[139] In fact, SARS-CoV-2 infection during pregnancy has been linked to numerous "adverse pregnancy outcomes including preeclampsia, preterm birth, and stillbirth."[140] For these reasons, pregnant women are particularly vulnerable to vaccine preventable diseases, while there is also no evidence of adverse outcomes from COVID-19 or other vaccines during pregnancy.[141]

Several vaccines are recommended for pregnant women, including COVID-19 shots as well as flu, pertussis and tetanus vaccines, because such diseases can cause severe illness and death in mothers, foetuses, and new-borns.[142] In fact, evidence has exposed how pregnant women and new-borns are particularly vulnerable to such diseases, though vaccines do not result in pregnancy complications.[143] Indeed, "Pregnant women were >4 times more likely to be hospitalised for novel influenza A (H1N1)-related complications than those infected in the general population, and accounted for 13% of all deaths from pandemic influenza A (H1N1)."[144] The rate of flu-related hospitalisations for healthy pregnant women is also 1 to 2 per 1000, which is 18 times greater than it is for healthy non-pregnant women.[145] Pregnant women are also in more danger of acute COVID-19 symptoms.[146] Such data continues to reveal that pregnant women can face staggeringly higher risks for severe illness, which is why public health experts have continued to urge expecting mothers to get vaccinated.

When it comes to trying to improve survival rates of mothers and their babies, vaccines are considered to be one of the safest and effective means of preventing deaths during and after pregnancy.[147] As Heidi Larson has sum-marised, "Maternal immunization is the missing link, adding to important existing antenatal interventions, to protect both mother and infant during some of the most vulnerable moments in both of their lives."[148] The WHO's Global Advisory Committee has outlined how this protection operates: "Maternal immunization can protect the mother directly against vaccine-preventable infections, and provide a cocooning effect that can potentially protect the fetus. It can also provide further direct fetal/infant protection against infection via the transport of specific antibodies to the fetus prior to birth."[149] Likewise, despite persuasive rumours, the WHO has found no evidence that vaccinating during pregnancy causes adverse effects. Numerous studies conducted from the 1960s onward, even through the COVID-19 pandemic, have collectively failed to identify harmful effects associated with vaccinating during pregnancy.[150] Instead, there are sig-nificant proven dangers for mothers and their children posed by vaccine preventable diseases.[151] Vaccination during pregnancy is safe, it is effective, and it is a powerful tool to save the lives of women and children across the globe. It is that safety factor, and the true risks for pregnant women *not* vaccinating, which must continually be communicated to the public in the face of the Danger theme in antivaccination messages.[152]

Danger and antivaccine persuasion

In 1956, one year after the virologist Jonas Salk announced that his team's polio vaccine had been successfully trialed, an Ohio cosmetics manufacturer named Duon Miller published an antivaccination pamphlet titled "'Fake' Polio Vaccine May Kill Your Child!"[153] Miller, who had previously been arrested on charges of mail fraud for spreading medical misinformation, founded *Polio Prevention Inc.* in Florida. Under this inscription, Miller dis-tributed counter-vaccine tracts across the country, and he spent years claiming that polio vaccines were injuring and killing countless children.[154] Miller's 1956 pamphlet is remarkable for a number of reasons. Firstly, it is hostile toward the polio vaccine. As this chapter has already identified, polio vaccines have been directly responsible for reducing poliomyelitis around the world. In the years before Miller's tract was published, the USA had experienced tens of thousands of new cases of polio per year, and the disease was a leading cause of disability and death in children. There was avid demand for a cure, and Jonas Salk became a national hero for pioneering an effective vaccine.[155] Hence, Miller's pamphlet was written when the severe effects of poliomyelitis were unmistakeable to America's public, and citizens were desperate for polio treatments.

Secondly, it is fascinating that this mid-20th century leaflet features many of the same persuasive cues and similar kinds of assertions as those observed in modern antivaccination messages. These include strident risk claims associated with the Danger theme, which are plainly voiced from the very start in the tract's title. This involves the Arousal of Fear persuasive cue, as it exclaims that the polio vaccine may kill readers' children. The tract goes on to insist, "All vaccines *against all diseases* have always left in their paths DEATH and ill health."[156] It asserts, "Vaccines have only filled countless cemeteries with innocent victims killed *prematurely* by FRAUDULENT injections." In the midst of such risk claims, Miller also employs the Asking Questions persuasive cue. "The 'promoters' of this dangerous vaccine give NO GUARANTEE or NO ASSURANCE that it will not KILL your child," contends the article. It then asks audiences, so "Why should you take a chance?" Miller further makes allegations which parallel the modern misunderstanding that vaccines are filled with deadly toxins. He advises readers to let "other callous parents permit this poisoning of their children," and warns: "One million little children will be offered as sacrifices on the altar of greed...having their life's blood '*polluted*' with Dr. Salk's fraudulent vaccine...dead virus '*pickled*' in formalin, (*formaldehyde*)...embalming fluid if you please." Using another rhetorical question, the pamphlet states that "they want to inject this 'embalming fluid' protein compound into the body of YOUR little child...*just how*LOW*can humans stoop?*" The article also echoes contemporary claims that vaccines can overload children's immune systems. "DON'T subject YOUR child's nervous system to the TERROR...SHOCK...and DANGEROUS result of this 'SERUM' injection *operation*," it cautions. Because the "sudden '*shock reaction*' following the injection of serums given to children is HORRIBLE!!'"

Along with such Danger messages the leaflet includes several accusations that correspond with the Distrust and Confidence motifs of antivaccine communications (Chapter 3). This involves the Scarcity Principle, expressed through numerous conspiratorial claims regarding the ineffectiveness of the polio vaccine being covered-up, and efforts "to prevent the public from learning the TRUTH." Miller's words also mirror the modern contention that vaccines are major money-makers. Accordingly, those promoting the vaccine are described as "unscrupulous '*money-grabbers*'," who "plan to inject this <u>unproven, unapproved, unscientific DANGEROUS</u>*vaccine* into the bodies of *little innocent children* for <u>NO REASON</u> in the world other than to protect their 'racket.'" The tract also references several doctors, who are apparently vehemently opposed to vaccination. In this way, it appeals to the credibility of medical specialists, while exemplifying the myth that research and experts discredit the scientific consensus. A doctor who is described as being famous is quoted as saying, "<u>vaccination is the cause of more disease</u> <u>and suffering than anything I could name</u>." All the while, statistics are thrown about, together with assertions that vaccines lead to numerous diseases, including those that they are intended to prevent. Miller assures readers that with vaccination there has occurred a "marked increase in the incidence of POLIO, <u>at least 400%</u>." In fact, "Statistics on this are so conclusive, no one can deny it." On top of that, the pamphlet espoused the myth that it was better sanitation and not vaccines that were truly responsible for reducing infectious diseases. "Smallpox and other plagues were eradicated by sanitation engineers," declared Miller, "<u>AFTER all</u> <u>*vaccines* and *serums* had FAILED COMPLETELY</u>."

Duon Miller's "'Fake' Polio Vaccine May Kill Your Child!" flyer encapsulates several key aspects of the DCD found in modern antivaccination communications. It also reveals how for decades many of the very same persuasive cues, and a variety of similar myths have been expressed in parallel ways by vaccine critics. Such tired claims have been applied to different vaccines over time, from polio to MMR, HPV and COVID-19, yet in each case they have been scientifically refuted. Nevertheless, they can still be persuasive when repackaged for modern audiences. Questions remain then whether, in a world impacted by consistent antivaccine persuasion motifs and persuasive cues, there are evidence-based approaches to reducing vaccine hesitancy and positively influencing people's vaccination behaviours? It is to such questions that the next two chapters turn, by considering vaccine advocacy tactics and techniques that have demonstrated the most promising results.

Notes

1 Benjamin Cunningham, "More Manic Than Movement," *The New Presence*, no. 3 (2010).
2 R. B. Aylward, "Eradicating Polio: Today's Challenges and Tomorrow's Legacy," *Annals of Tropical Medicine & Parasitology* 100, no. 5–6 (2006): 402.
3 Adapted from ibid.
4 Adapted from ibid.
5 Matthew Janko, "Vaccination: A Victim of Its Own Success," *Virtual Mentor* 14, no. 1 (2012).
6 David Butler Jones, quoted in Christopher J. Rutty et al., *Conquering the Crippler: Canada and the Eradication of Polio* (Ottawa: Canadian Public Health Association, 2005), 3.

7 Stephanie L. Enkel et al., "'Hesitant Compliers': Qualitative Analysis of Concerned Fully-Vaccinating Parents," *Vaccine* 36, no. 44 (2018); P. H. Streefland, A. M. Chowdhury, and P. Ramos-Jimenez, "Quality of Vaccination Services and Social Demand for Vaccinations in Africa and Asia," *Bulletin of the World Health Organization* 77, no. 9 (1999); Mabel Berezin and Alicia Eads, "Risk Is for the Rich? Childhood Vaccination Resistance and a Culture of Health," *Social Science & Medicine* 165 (2016).

8 E. J. Gangarosa et al., "Impact of Anti-Vaccine Movements on Pertussis Control: The Untold Story," *Lancet* 351, no. 9099 (1998).

9 Ibid., 360.

10 Andrea Stöckl and Anna Smajdor, "The MMR Debate in the United Kingdom: Vaccine Scare, Statesmanship and the Media," in *The Politics of Vaccination: A Global History*, ed. Christine Holmberg, Stuart Blume, and Paul Greenough (Manchester: Manchester University Press, 2017).

11 David C. Burgess, Margaret A. Burgess, and Julie Leask, "The MMR Vaccination and Autism Controversy in United Kingdom 1998–2005: Inevitable Community Outrage or a Failure of Risk Communication?," *Vaccine* 24, no. 18 (2006): 3921.

12 WHO, "Human Papillomavirus (HPV) and Cervical Cancer," World Health Organization, https://www.who.int/news-room/fact-sheets/detail/human-papillomavirus-(hpv)-and-cervical-cancer.

13 Neil Durham, "British Schoolgirl Dies after Receiving HPV Vaccine," GP, https://www.gponline.com/british-schoolgirl-dies-receiving-hpv-vaccine/article/941663.

14 Adrian O'Dowd, "Teenager Who Died after Having HPV Vaccine Had a Malignant Chest Tumour," *BMJ* 339 (2009): 1.

15 Michael Hiltzik, "How a Major Newspaper Bungled a Vaccine Story, Then Smeared Its Critics," *Los Angeles Times*, https://www.latimes.com/business/hiltzik/la-fi-mh-how-a-major-newspaper-20150213-column.html.

16 L. Arnheim-Dahlstrom et al., "Autoimmune, Neurological, and Venous Thromboembolic Adverse Events after Immunisation of Adolescent Girls with Quadrivalent Human Papillomavirus Vaccine in Denmark and Sweden: Cohort Study," *BMJ* 347, no. 4 (2013): 4.

17 Brenda Corcoran, Anna Clarke, and Tom Barrett, "Rapid Response to HPV Vaccination Crisis in Ireland," *Lancet* 391, no. 10135 (2018); Camilla Hiul Suppli et al., "Decline in HPV-Vaccination Uptake in Denmark – the Association between HPV-Related Media Coverage and HPV-Vaccination," *BMC Public Health* 18, no. 1 (2018).

18 "Parents Are Taking Desperate Measures Because of Government Discrimination," AVN, https://avn.org.au/2016/03/parents-taking-desperate-measures-government-discrimination/; "Media Release – a New Billboard Gives a Voice to the Vaccine Injured," AVN, https://avn.org.au/2017/11/16262/; Meghan Bridgid Moran et al., "What Makes Anti-Vaccine Websites Persuasive? A Content Analysis of Techniques Used by Anti-Vaccine Websites to Engender Anti-Vaccine Sentiment," *Journal of Communication in Healthcare* 9, no. 3 (2016).

19 "Injected and Neglected – Irish Gardasil Protest," AVN, https://avn.org.au/2018/07/injected-and-neglected-irish-gardasil-protest/.

20 "Claims Vaccines Do Not Cause Autism Have No Substance, an Australian Perspective – Part 2," AVN, https://avn.org.au/2019/04/claims-vaccines-do-not-cause-autism-have-no-substance-an-australian-perspective-part-2/; John Piesse, "Vaccines Are Unavoidably Unsafe – by Dr John Piesse," AVN, https://avn.org.au/2017/08/vaccines-unavoidably-unsafe-dr-john-piesse/.

21 Tasha David, "There Is Nothing Trendy About Not Vaccinating Your Child," AVN, https://avn.org.au/2018/08/there-is-nothing-trendy-about-not-vaccinating-your-child/.

22 Michael Belkin, "Vaccine-Related Death – Lyla Rose," AVN, https://avn.org.au/2012/04/died-from-vaccines-lyla-rose/.

23 "Under the Wire Episode 6, September 7, 2019," https://avn.org.au/2019/09/under-the-wire-episode-6-september-7-2019/.

24 Faith Gleicher and Richard E. Petty, "Expectations of Reassurance Influence the Nature of Fear-Stimulated Attitude Change," *Journal of Experimental Social Psychology* 28 (1992).

25 Jonah Berger, "Arousal Increases Social Transmission of Information," *Psychological Science* 22, no. 7 (2011).

26 Dan M. Kahan, "Two Conceptions of Emotion in Risk Regulation," *University of Pennsylvania Law Review* 156, no. 3 (2008).

27 Anna Winterbottom et al., "Does Narrative Information Bias Individual's Decision Making? A Systematic Review," *Social Science & Medicine* 67, no. 12 (2008).

28 Cornelia Betsch et al., "Opportunities and Challenges of Web 2.0 for Vaccination Decisions," *Vaccine* 30, no. 25 (2012).

29 Amanda Hinnant, Roma Subramanian, and Rachel Young, "User Comments on Climate Stories: Impacts of Anecdotal Vs. Scientific Evidence," *An Interdisciplinary, International Journal Devoted to the Description, Causes and Implications of Climatic Change* 138, no. 3–4 (2016): 413.

30 Abdulmaged M. Traish, Jay C. Vance, and Abraham Morgentaler, "Overselling Hysteria," *EMBO Reports* 18, no. 1 (2017): 15.

31 "Vaccine-Injured – Robert," AVN, https://avn.org.au/2012/04/vaccine-injured-robert/; Brian Hughes et al., "Development of a Codebook of Online Anti-Vaccination Rhetoric to Manage COVID-19 Vaccine Misinformation," *International Journal of Environmental Research and Public Health* 18, no. 14 (2021).

32 "Chief Medical Officer Admits Whooping Cough Lies Informed No Jab No Pay/Play," AVN, https://avn.org.au/2018/09/cmo-admits-whooping-cough-lies-informed-no-jab-pay-play/.

33 "Time for a Wide-Ranging & Independent Inquiry into the Effectiveness and Safety of Vaccination," AVN, https://avn.org.au/2017/03/time-wide-ranging-independent-inquiry-effectiveness-safety-vaccination/.

34 Tasha David, "Modern Day Zealots with a Pen," AVN, https://avn.org.au/2016/03/6543/.

35 Thomas Aechtner, *Media and the Science-Religion Conflict: Mass Persuasion in the Evolution Wars* (Abingdon: Routledge, 2020), 137–39.

36 Don Reisinger, "A Look Back at Steve Jobs and Apple's 'Get a Mac' Ads," Fortune, http://fortune.com/2016/12/09/apple-get-a-mac-ads/.

37 Randall Livingstone, "Better at Life Stuff: Consumption, Identity, and Class in Apple's 'Get a Mac' Campaign,' *The Journal of Communication Inquiry* 35, no. 3 (2011): 218.

38 Darreld Muehling, Jeffrey Stoltman, and Sanford Grossbart, "The Impact of Comparative Advertising on Levels of Message Involvement," *Journal of Advertising* 19, no. 4 (1990); Dhruv Grewal et al., "Comparative Versus Noncomparative Advertising: A Meta-Analysis," *Journal of Marketing* 61, no. 4 (1997).

39 Alan T. Shao, Yeqing Bao, and Elizabeth Gray, "Comparative Advertising Effectiveness: A Cross-Cultural Study," *Journal of Current Issues & Research in Advertising* 26, no. 2 (2004); Enrique Manzur et al., "Comparative Advertising

Effectiveness in Latin America: Evidence from Chile," *International Marketing Review* 29, no. 3 (2012): 278.

40 Robert B. Cialdini, *Influence: Science and Practice*, 5th ed. (Boston: Pearson Education, 2009), 12.

41 Ibid., 13.

42 Cornelia Pechmann and Gabriel Esteban, "Persuasion Processes Associated with Direct Comparative and Noncomparative Advertising and Implications for Advertising Effectiveness," *Journal of Consumer Psychology* 2, no. 4 (1993).

43 Karen E. James and Paul J. Hensel, "Negative Advertising: The Malicious Strain of Comparative Advertising," *Journal of Advertising* 20, no. 2 (1991).

44 Ross D. Petty and Paul M. Spink, "Comparative Advertising Law in the European Community: Will the Proposed Directive Harmonize across the Atlantic?," *Journal of Public Policy & Marketing* 14, no. 2 (1995); Francesca Barigozzi and Martin Peitz, "Comparative Advertising and Competition Policy," *Alma Mater Digital Library, Universita di Balogna* (2004), http://amsacta. cib.unibo.it/1563/1/524.pdf.

45 Alinab Sorescu and Betsyd Gelb, "Negative Comparative Advertising: Evidence Favoring Fine-Tuning," *Journal of Advertising* 29, no. 4 (2000).

46 George Y. Bizer and Richard E. Petty, "How We Conceptualize Our Attitudes Matters: The Effects of Valence Framing on the Resistance of Political Attitudes," *Political Psychology* 26, no. 4 (2005): 554.

47 Ibid., 554–55.

48 L. F. Vernon, "Is Vaccine Dissent Based on Science?," *Health Education and Care* 2, no. 4 (2017); Michael Eisenstein, "Public Health: An Injection of Trust," *Nature* 507, no. 7490 (2014).

49 "Autism and Vaccines," Centers for Disease Control and Prevention, https:// www.cdc.gov/vaccinesafety/concerns/autism.html.

50 "What Is Autism Spectrum Disorder?," Centers for Disease Control and Prevention, https://www.cdc.gov/ncbddd/autism/facts.html.

51 A. J. Wakefield et al., "Ileal-Lymphoid-Nodular Hyperplasia, Non-Specific Colitis, and Pervasive Developmental Disorder in Children," *Lancet* 351, no. 9103 (1998).

52 Brian Deer, *The Doctor Who Fooled the World: Andrew Wakefield's War on Vaccines* (Brunswick: Scribe Publications, 2020).

53 Fiona Godlee, Jane Smith, and Harvey Marcovitch, "Wakefield's Article Linking MMR Vaccine and Autism Was Fraudulent," *BMJ* 342, no. 1 (2011).

54 G. Baird, A. Pickles, and E. Simonoff, "Measles Vaccination and Antibody Response in Autism Spectrum Disorders," *Archives of Disease in Childhood* 93, no. 10 (2008); C. Black, J. Kaye, and H. Jick, "Relation of Childhood Gastrointestinal Disorders to Autism: Nested Case-Control Study Using Data from the UK General Practice Research Database," *BMJ* 325, no. 7361 (2002); W. Chen et al., "No Evidence for Links between Autism, MMR and Measles Virus," *Psychological Medicine* 34, no. 3 (2004); Loring Dales, Sandra Jo Hammer, and Natalie J. Smith, "Time Trends in Autism and in MMR Immunization Coverage in California," *JAMA* 285, no. 9 (2001); Robert L. Davis et al., "Measles-Mumps-Rubella and Other Measles-Containing Vaccines Do Not Increase the Risk for Inflammatory Bowel Disease: A Case-Control Study from the Vaccine Safety Datalink Project," *Archives of Pediatrics & Adolescent Medicine* 155, no. 3 (2001); Frank Destefano et al., "Age at First Measles-Mumps-Rubella Vaccination in Children with Autism and School-Matched Control Subjects: A Population-Based Study in Metropolitan Atlanta," *Pediatrics* 113, no. 2 (2004); A. Doja and W. Roberts, "Immunizations and Autism: A Review of the Literature," *Canadian Journal of Neurological Sciences* 33, no. 4 (2006); Yasmin D'Souza, Eric Fombonne, and Brian J.

Ward, "No Evidence of Persisting Measles Virus in Peripheral Blood Mononuclear Cells from Children with Autism Spectrum Disorder (Testing)," *Pediatrics* 118, no. 4 (2006); C. Paddy Farrington, Elizabeth Miller, and Brent Taylor, "MMR and Autism: Further Evidence against a Causal Association," *Vaccine* 19, no. 27 (2001); Eric Fombonne and Suniti Chakrabarti, "No Evidence for a New Variant of Measles-Mumps-Rubella-Induced Autism," *Pediatrics* 108, no. 4 (2001); Eric Fombonne et al., "Pervasive Developmental Disorders in Montreal, Quebec, Canada: Prevalence and Links with Immunizations," *Pediatrics* 118, no. 1 (2006); Hideo Honda, Yasuo Shimizu, and Michael Rutter, "No Effect of MMR Withdrawal on the Incidence of Autism: A Total Population Study," *Journal of Child Psychology and Psychiatry* 46, no. 6 (2005); Mady Hornig et al., "Lack of Association between Measles Virus Vaccine and Autism with Enteropathy: A Case-Control Study," *PLoS One* 3, no. 9 (2008); IOM, *Immunization Safety Review: Vaccines and Autism*, Vaccines and Autism (Washington, D.C.: National Academies Press, 2004); Anjali Jain et al., "Autism Occurrence by MMR Vaccine Status among US Children with Older Siblings with and without Autism," *JAMA* 313, no. 15 (2015); Ja Kaye, M. Del Mar Melero-Montes, and H. Jick, "Mumps, Measles, and Rubella Vaccine and the Incidence of Autism Recorded by General Practitioners: A Time Trend Analysis," *BMJ* 322, no. 7281 (2001); Kristin C. Klein and Emily B. Diehl, "Relationship between MMR Vaccine and Autism," *Annals of Pharmacotherapy* 38, no. 7–8 (2004); R. Lingam et al., "Prevalence of Autism and Parentally Reported Triggers in a North East London Population," *Archives of Disease in Childhood* 88, no. 8 (2003); Kreesten Meldgaard Madsen et al., "A Population-Based Study of Measles, Mumps, and Rubella Vaccination and Autism," *The New England Journal of Medicine* 347, no. 19 (2002); Annamari Makela, J. Nuorti, and Heikki Peltola, "Neurologic Disorders after Measles-Mumps-Rebella Vaccination," *Pediatrics* 110, no. 5 (2002); Dorota Mrożek-Budzyn, Agnieszka Kiełtyka, and Renata Majewska, "Lack of Association between Measles-Mumps-Rubella Vaccination and Autism in Children: A Case-Control Study," *The Pediatric Infectious Disease Journal* 29, no. 5 (2010); Heikki Peltola et al., "No Evidence for Measles, Mumps, and Rubella Vaccine-Associated Inflammatory Bowel Disease or Autism in a 14-Year Prospective Study," *Lancet* 351, no. 9112 (1998); Jennifer Richler et al., "Is There a 'Regressive Phenotype' of Autism Spectrum Disorder Associated with the Measles-Mumps-Rubella Vaccine? A CPEA Study," *Journal of Autism and Developmental Disorders* 36, no. 3 (2006); Liam Smeeth et al., "MMR Vaccination and Pervasive Developmental Disorders: A Case-Control Study," *Lancet* 364, no. 9438 (2004); B. Taylor et al., "Autism and Measles, Mumps, and Rubella Vaccine: No Epidemiological Evidence for a Causal Association," *Lancet* 353, no. 9169 (1999); Brent Taylor et al., "Measles, Mumps, and Rubella Vaccination and Bowel Problems or Developmental Regression in Children with Autism: Population Study," *BMJ* 324, no. 7334 (2002); Tokio Uchiyama, Michiko Kurosawa, and Yutaka Inaba, "MMR-Vaccine and Regression in Autism Spectrum Disorders: Negative Results Presented from Japan," *Journal of Autism and Developmental Disorders* 37, no. 2 (2007).

55   David Cohen et al., "Specific Genetic Disorders and Autism: Clinical Contribution Towards Their Identification," *Journal of Autism and Developmental Disorders* 35, no. 1 (2005); Jacob A. S. Vorstman et al., "Autism Genetics: Opportunities and Challenges for Clinical Translation," *Nature Reviews Genetics* 18, no. 6 (2017); Holly A. F. Stessman et al., "Targeted Sequencing Identifies 91 Neurodevelopmental-Disorder Risk Genes with Autism and Developmental-Disability Biases," *Nature Genetics* 49, no. 4 (2017); M. S.

Durkin et al., "Advanced Parental Age and the Risk of Autism Spectrum Disorder," *American Journal of Epidemiology* 168, no. 11 (2008); S. Wu et al., "Advanced Parental Age and Autism Risk in Children: A Systematic Review and Meta-Analysis," *Acta Psychiatrica Scandinavica* 135, no. 1 (2017).

56 H. Gardener, D. Spiegelman, and S. L. Buka, "Perinatal and Neonatal Risk Factors for Autism: A Comprehensive Meta-Analysis," *Pediatrics* 128, no. 2 (2011).

57 Jeffrey S. Gerber and Paul A. Offit, "Vaccines and Autism: A Tale of Shifting Hypotheses," *Clinical Infectious Diseases* 48, no. 4 (2009).

58 Katrina F. Brown et al., "UK Parents' Decision-Making About Measles–Mumps–Rubella (MMR) Vaccine 10 Years after the MMR-Autism Controversy: A Qualitative Analysis," *Vaccine* 30, no. 10 (2012).

59 S. Koppen et al., "No Epidemiological Evidence for Infant Vaccinations to Cause Allergic Disease," *Vaccine* 22, no. 25 (2004).

60 H. Okada et al., "The 'Hygiene Hypothesis' for Autoimmune and Allergic Diseases: An Update," *Clinical and Experimental Immunology* 160, no. 1 (2010): 1.

61 Koppen et al., "No Epidemiological Evidence for Infant Vaccinations to Cause Allergic Disease," 3375.

62 Ibid.

63 Thomas A. E. Platts-Mills, "The Allergy Epidemics: 1870–2010," *The Journal of Allergy and Clinical Immunology* 136, no. 1 (2015): 9.

64 Ibid.

65 Megan Scudellari, "News Feature: Cleaning up the Hygiene Hypothesis," *Proceedings of the National Academy of Sciences USA* 114, no. 7 (2017).

66 "AVN Leaflet," AVN, https://avn.org.au/leaflet/.

67 Ibid.

68 Lucija Tomljenovic, "Forced Vaccinations: For the Greater Good?," *The Vaccine Choice Journal* Special Supplement (2015): 10.

69 Koppen et al., "No Epidemiological Evidence for Infant Vaccinations to Cause Allergic Disease," 1.

70 Erika von Mutius, "Allergies, Infections and the Hygiene Hypothesis – the Epidemiological Evidence," *Immunobiology* 212, no. 6 (2007): 436.

71 Ibid.

72 Franz E. Babl, Stuart Lewena, and Lance Brown, "Vaccination-Related Adverse Events," *Pediatric Emergency Care* 22, no. 7 (2006): 515.

73 Julia M. L. Brotherton et al., "Anaphylaxis Following Quadrivalent Human Papillomavirus Vaccination," *CMAJ* 179, no. 6 (2008).

74 Peter Adams, "What Are the Chances of Being Struck by Lightning?," 9News, https://www.9news.com.au/national/what-are-the-chances-of-being-struck-by-lightning/00f73a30-01f3-407d-a368-c9f75f2cad91.

75 David C. Wraith, Michel Goldman, and Paul-Henri Lambert, "Vaccination and Autoimmune Disease: What Is the Evidence?," *Lancet* 362, no. 9396 (2003): 1659.

76 Jean-François Bach, "The Effect of Infections on Susceptibility to Autoimmune and Allergic Diseases," *N Engl J Med* 347, no. 12 (2002).

77 "Debunked: ABC News | Flu Shot More Likely to Save Your Life Than Not Getting It, Says Influenza Researcher, 08 August 2019," AVN, https://avn.org.au/vaccination-media-watch/rebuttal-abc-news-flu-shot-more-likely-to-save-your-life-than-not-getting-it-says-influenza-researcher/.

78 "The Gardasil Vaccine – Bad Science, Great Promotion, Dangerous," AVN, https://avn.org.au/2018/05/gardasil-vaccine-bad-science-great-promotion-dangerous/.

79 Robert T. Chen, Robert Pless, and Frank Destefano, "Epidemiology of Autoimmune Reactions Induced by Vaccination," *J Autoimmun* 16, no. 3 (2001).

80 "Guillain-Barré Syndrome," National Institute of Neurological Disorders and Stroke, https://www.ninds.nih.gov/health-information/disorders/guillain-barre-syndrome.

81 S. K. Greene et al., "Risk of Confirmed Guillain-Barre Syndrome Following Receipt of Monovalent Inactivated Influenza a (H1N1) and Seasonal Influenza Vaccines in the Vaccine Safety Datalink Project, 2009–2010," *American Journal of Epidemiology* 175, no. 11 (2012).

82 Daniel A. Salmon et al., "Association between Guillain-Barré Syndrome and Influenza a (H1N1) 2009 Monovalent Inactivated Vaccines in the USA: A Meta-Analysis," *Lancet* 381, no. 9876 (2013): 1465.

83 Wraith, Goldman, and Lambert, "Vaccination and Autoimmune Disease: What Is the Evidence?," 1663.

84 Sharon K. Greene et al., "Guillain-Barré Syndrome, Influenza Vaccination, and Antecedent Respiratory and Gastrointestinal Infections: A Case-Centered Analysis in the Vaccine Safety Datalink, 2009–2011," *PLoS One* 8, no. 6 (2013); A. T. Kawai et al., "Absence of Associations between Influenza Vaccines and Increased Risks of Seizures, Guillain-Barré Syndrome, Encephalitis, or Anaphylaxis in the 2012–2013 Season," *Pharmacoepidemiology and Drug Safety* 23, no. 5 (2014); Baxter Roger et al., "Recurrent Guillain-Barré Syndrome Following Vaccination," *Clinical Infectious Diseases* 54, no. 6 (2012).

85 C. R. Simpson et al., "First-Dose Chadox1 and Bnt162b2 COVID-19 Vaccines and Thrombocytopenic, Thromboembolic and Hemorrhagic Events in Scotland," *Nature Medicine* 27, no. 7 (2021); Colin R. Simpson et al., "Second-Dose Chadox1 and Bnt162b2 COVID-19 Vaccines and Thrombocytopenic, Thromboembolic and Hemorrhagic Events in Scotland," *Nature Communications* 13, no. 1 (2022); A. K. Ghosh et al., "Bnt162b2 COVID-19 Vaccine Induced Immune Thrombocytopenic Purpura," *Case Reports in Medicine* 2022 (2022); Luna Vorster et al., "Covid-19 Vaccine (mRNA Bnt162b2) and Covid-19 Infection-Induced Thrombotic Thrombocytopenic Purpura in Adolescents," *Pediatric Blood & Cancer* 69, no. 6 (2022); Finn-Ole Paulsen et al., "Immune Thrombocytopenic Purpura after Vaccination with COVID-19 Vaccine (Chadox1 Ncov-19)," *Blood* 138, no. 11 (2021); Hiroaki Akiyama et al., "Immune Thrombocytopenia Associated with Pfizer-Biontech's Bnt162b2 mRNA COVID-19 Vaccine," *IDCases* 25 (2021).

86 "Idiopathic Thrombocytopenic Purpura," Johns Hopkins Medicine, https://www.hopkinsmedicine.org/health/conditions-and-diseases/idiopathic-thrombocytopenic-purpura

87 Elpis Mantadakis, Evangelia Farmaki, and George R. Buchanan, "Thrombocytopenic Purpura after Measles-Mumps-Rubella Vaccination: A Systematic Review of the Literature and Guidance for Management," *Journal of Pediatrics* 156, no. 4 (2010): 623.

88 Wraith, Goldman, and Lambert, "Vaccination and Autoimmune Disease: What Is the Evidence?," 1663.

89 S. Bhattacharjee and M. Banerjee, "Immune Thrombocytopenia Secondary to COVID-19: A Systematic Review," *SN Comprehensive Clinical Medicine* 2, no. 11 (2020); M. G. Alharbi et al., "COVID-19 Associated with Immune Thrombocytopenia: A Systematic Review and Meta-Analysis," *Expert Review of Hematology* 15, no. 2 (2022); R. Root-Bernstein, J. Huber, and A. Ziehl, "Complementary Sets of Autoantibodies Induced by SARS-CoV-2, Adenovirus and Bacterial Antigens Cross-React with Human Blood Protein Antigens in COVID-19 Coagulopathies," *International Journal of Molecular Sciences* 23, no. 19 (2022); Hiroto Kaneko et al., "Relapse of Idiopathic Thrombocytopenic Purpura Caused by Influenza a Virus Infection: A Case Report," *Journal of Infection and Chemotherapy* 10, no. 6 (2004).

90 Julia Hippisley-Cox et al., "Risk of Thrombocytopenia and Thromboembolism after Covid-19 Vaccination and SARS-CoV-2 Positive Testing: Self-Controlled Case Series Study," *BMJ* 374 (2021); Elpis Mantadakis et al., "A Case of Immune Thrombocytopenic Purpura after Influenza Vaccination: Consequence or Coincidence?," *Journal of Pediatric Hematology/Oncology* 32, no. 6 (2010).

91 Martina Patone et al., "Risks of Myocarditis, Pericarditis, and Cardiac Arrhythmias Associated with COVID-19 Vaccination or SARS-CoV-2 Infection," *Nature Medicine* 28, no. 2 (2022).

92 Tegan K. Boehmer et al., "Association between COVID-19 and Myocarditis Using Hospital-Based Administrative Data – United States, March 2020–January 2021," *Morbidity and Mortality Weekly Report* 70, no. 35 (2021); Navya Voleti, Surya Prakash Reddy, and Paddy Ssentongo, "Myocarditis in SARS-CoV-2 Infection Vs. COVID-19 Vaccination: A Systematic Review and Meta-Analysis," *Frontiers in Cardiovascular Medicine* 9 (2022); Jennifer Abbasi, "The Covid Heart – One Year after SARS-CoV-2 Infection, Patients Have an Array of Increased Cardiovascular Risks," *JAMA* 327, no. 12 (2022).

93 Brendan Kergin, "Several Hundred Show up to Vancouver Protest of Bill Gates (Photos)," Vancouver is Awesome, https://www.vmcdn.ca/f/files/via/images/politics-local/cairnse-superprotest-04-10-22-5036.jpg;w=960;h=640;bgcolor=000000.

94 Fergus Hunter, "Third Day of Charges at Bowral Organic Food Store over COVID-19 Breaches," *Sydney Morning Herald*, https://www.smh.com.au/national/nsw/wacko-views-third-day-of-charges-at-bowral-organic-food-store-over-covid-19-breaches-20210703-p586jo.html.

95 William T. Shearer et al., "Recommendations for Live Viral and Bacterial Vaccines in Immunodeficient Patients and Their Close Contacts," *Journal of Allergy and Clinical Immunology* 133, no. 4 (2014).

96 Evan J. Dr Anderson, "Rotavirus Vaccines: Viral Shedding and Risk of Transmission," *Lancet* 8, no. 10 (2008); H. C. Sachs, "The Transfer of Drugs and Therapeutics into Human Breast Milk: An Update on Selected Topics," *Pediatrics* 132, no. 3 (2013).

97 "Chickenpox (Varicella) Vaccines," Centers for Disease Control and Prevention, https://www.cdc.gov/vaccinesafety/vaccines/varicella-vaccine.html.

98 Lee M. Hampton et al., "Cessation of Trivalent Oral Poliovirus Vaccine and Introduction of Inactivated Poliovirus Vaccine – Worldwide, 2016," *MMWR: Morbidity and Mortality Weekly Report* 65, no. 35 (2016).

99 "Poliomyelitis," World Health Organization, https://www.who.int/teams/health-product-policy-and-standards/standards-and-specifications/vaccines-quality/poliomyelitis.

100 "IPV," Global Polio Eradication Initiative, http://polioeradication.org/polio-today/polio-prevention/the-vaccines/ipv/.

101 P. E. Fine and I. A. Carneiro, "Transmissibility and Persistence of Oral Polio Vaccine Viruses: Implications for the Global Poliomyelitis Eradication Initiative," *American Journal of Epidemiology* 150, no. 10 (1999).

102 "What Is Vaccine-Derived Polio?," https://www.who.int/news-room/q-a-detail/what-is-vaccine-derived-polio.

103 Ibid.

104 "Chickenpox and Shingles Fact Sheet," NSW Government, https://www.health.nsw.gov.au/Infectious/factsheets/Pages/chickenpox.aspx; Ulrich Heininger and Jane F. Seward, "Varicella," *Lancet* 368, no. 9544 (2006).

105 Tara C. Smith, "Vaccine Rejection and Hesitancy: A Review and Call to Action," *Open Forum Infectious Diseases* 4, no. 3 (2017): 1–2; Anna Kata, "A

Postmodern Pandora's Box: Anti-Vaccination Misinformation on the Internet," *Vaccine* 28, no. 7 (2010): 1711.

106   Patrick Davies, Simon Chapman, and Julie Leask, "Antivaccination Activists on the World Wide Web," *Archives of Disease in Childhood* 87, no. 1 (2002): 23.

107   "Common Ingredients in U.S. Licensed Vaccines," Food & Drug Administration, https://www.fda.gov/vaccines-blood-biologics/safety-availability-biologics/common-ingredients-us-licensed-vaccines.

108   Adapted from Paul Stehr-Green et al., "Autism and Thimerosal-Containing Vaccines: Lack of Consistent Evidence for an Association," *American Journal of Preventive Medicine* 25, no. 2 (2003): 104.

109   Michael E. Pichichero et al., "Mercury Concentrations and Metabolism in Infants Receiving Vaccines Containing Thiomersal: A Descriptive Study," *Lancet* 360, no. 9347 (2002).

110   Stehr-Green et al., "Autism and Thimerosal-Containing Vaccines: Lack of Consistent Evidence for an Association."; K. M. Madsen et al., "Thimerosal and the Occurrence of Autism: Negative Ecological Evidence from Danish Population-Based Data," *Pediatrics* 112, no. 3 (2003); Anders Hviid et al., "Association between Thimerosal-Containing Vaccine and Autism," *JAMA* 290, no. 13 (2003).

111   N. Andrews, "Thimerosal Exposure in Infants and Developmental Disorders: A Retrospective Cohort Study in the United Kingdom Does Not Support a Causal Association," *Pediatrics* 114, no. 3 (2004); Jon Heron, Jean Golding, and Alspac Study Team and, "Thimerosal Exposure in Infants and Developmental Disorders: A Prospective Cohort Study in the United Kingdom Does Not Support a Causal Association," *Pediatrics*; William W. Thompson et al., "Early Thimerosal Exposure and Neuropsychological Outcomes at 7 to 10 Years," *New England Journal of Medicine* 357, no. 13 (2007).

112   Michael Shevell and Eric Fombonne, "Autism and MMR Vaccination or Thimerosal Exposure: An Urban Legend?," *Canadian Journal of Neurological Sciences* 33, no. 4 (2006): 339.

113   Meryl Dorey, "Why the Avn?."

114   Thomas Aechtner, "Distrust, Danger, and Confidence: A Content Analysis of the Australian Vaccination-Risks Network Blog," *Public Understanding of Science* (2020).

115   "Darwin-Skeptic Mass Media: Examining Persuasion in the Evolution Wars," *Journal of Media and Religion* 13, no. 4 (2014): 192.

116   Richard A. Lanham, *A Handlist of Rhetorical Terms*, 2nd ed. (London: University of California Press, 1991), 9–10, 71, 87.

117   Jon Scott Armstrong, *Persuasive Advertising Evidence-Based Principles* (Basingstoke: Palgrave Macmillan, 2010), 166.

118   Richard E. Petty and John T. Cacioppo, *Communication and Persuasion: Central and Peripheral Routes to Attitude Change* (New York: Springer-Verlag, 1986), 198–203.

119   Rohini Ahluwalia and Robert E. Burnkrant, "Answering Questions About Questions: A Persuasion Knowledge Perspective for Understanding the Effects of Rhetorical Questions," *Journal of Consumer Research* 31, no. 1 (2004): 27.

120   "Flu Shots Should Be Mandatory for Hospital Workers: CMAJ | CTV News," AVN, https://avn.org.au/2012/10/flu-shots-should-be-mandatory-for-hospital-workers-cmaj-ctv-news/; "Challenging Conflicts of Interest in Coercive Vaccination Policy," AVN, https://avn.org.au/2019/05/challenging-conflicts-of-interest-in-coercive-vaccination-policy/; "No Link between Measles Vaccine and Autism – Not True," https://avn.org.au/2019/03/no-link-between-measles-vaccine-and-autism-not-true/.

121 "Safety of Aluminium in Vaccines: NCIRS vs Professor Chris Exley," AVN, https://avn.org.au/2019/11/safety-of-aluminium-in-vaccines-ncirs-vs-professor-chris-exley/; Robert M. Wolfe, "Vaccine Safety Activists on the Internet," *Expert Review of Vaccines* 1, no. 3 (2002); Donald C. Arthur, "Negative Portrayal of Vaccines by Commercial Websites: Tortious Misrepresentation," *UMass Law Review* 11, no. 2 (2016).

122 Davies, Chapman, and Leask, "Antivaccination Activists on the World Wide Web."

123 David, "There Is Nothing Trendy About Not Vaccinating Your Child".

124 Aechtner, "Darwin-Skeptic Mass Media: Examining Persuasion in the Evolution Wars"; Allison Kennedy et al., "Confidence About Vaccines in the United States: Understanding Parents' Perceptions," *Health Affairs* 30, no. 6 (2011).

125 Smith, "Vaccine Rejection and Hesitancy: A Review and Call to Action," 2; Nathan J. Rodriguez, "Vaccine-Hesitant Justifications: 'Too Many, Too Soon,' Narrative Persuasion, and the Conflation of Expertise," *Global Qualitative Nursing Research* 3 (2016): 5; A. Kennedy, M. Basket, and K. Sheedy, "Vaccine Attitudes, Concerns, and Information Sources Reported by Parents of Young Children: Results from the 2009 Healthstyles Survey," *Pediatrics* 127, no. Supplement (2011): 94; Bruce G. Gellin, Edward W. Maibach, and Edgar K. Marcuse, "Do Parents Understand Immunizations? A National Telephone Survey," *Pediatrics* 106, no. 5 (2000).

126 Belkin, "Vaccine-Related Death – Lyla Rose".

127 Jason M. Glanz et al., "Association between Estimated Cumulative Vaccine Antigen Exposure through the First 23 Months of Life and Non-Vaccine-Targeted Infections from 24 through 47 Months of Age," *JAMA* 319, no. 9 (2018): 907.

128 Gerber and Offit, "Vaccines and Autism: A Tale of Shifting Hypotheses," 460.

129 P. A. Offit et al., "Addressing Parents' Concerns: Do Multiple Vaccines Overwhelm or Weaken the Infant's Immune System?," *Pediatrics* 109, no. 1 (2002): 126.

130 Ibid.

131 Glanz et al., "Association between Estimated Cumulative Vaccine Antigen Exposure through the First 23 Months of Life and Non–Vaccine-Targeted Infections from 24 through 47 Months of Age."

132 M. J. Smith and C. R. Woods, "On-Time Vaccine Receipt in the First Year Does Not Adversely Affect Neuropsychological Outcomes," *Pediatrics* 125, no. 6 (2010).

133 Jason M. Glanz et al., "Association between Undervaccination with Diphtheria, Tetanus Toxoids, and Acellular Pertussis (DTaP) Vaccine and Risk of Pertussis Infection in Children 3 to 36 Months of Age," *JAMA Pediatrics* 167, no. 11 (2013).

134 S. Otto et al., "General Non-Specific Morbidity Is Reduced after Vaccination within the Third Month of Life – the Greifswald Study," *Journal of Infection* 41, no. 2 (2000): 172.

135 Frank DeStefano, Cristofer S. Price, and Eric S. Weintraub, "Increasing Exposure to Antibody-Stimulating Proteins and Polysaccharides in Vaccines Is Not Associated with Risk of Autism," *Journal of Pediatrics* 163, no. 2 (2013): 563.

136 Sam Martin et al., ""Vaccines for Pregnant Women...?! Absurd' – Mapping Maternal Vaccination Discourse and Stance on Social Media over Six Months," *Vaccine* 38, no. 42 (2020); Christopher R. Wilcox et al., "Influenza and Pertussis Vaccination in Pregnancy: Portrayal in Online Media Articles and Perceptions of Pregnant Women and Healthcare Professionals," *Vaccine* 36, no. 50 (2018).

137   Milad Azami et al., "COVID-19 Vaccine Acceptance among Pregnant Women Worldwide: A Systematic Review and Meta-Analysis," *PLoS One* 17, no. 9 (2022); Petros Galanis et al., "Uptake of COVID-19 Vaccines among Pregnant Women: A Systematic Review and Meta-Analysis," *Vaccines* 10, no. 5 (2022); V. Male, "Are COVID-19 Vaccines Safe in Pregnancy?," *Nature Reviews Immunology* 21, no. 4 (2021).

138   Martin et al., "'Vaccines for Pregnant Women...?! Absurd' – Mapping Maternal Vaccination Discourse and Stance on Social Media over Six Months," 6634.

139   Rose J. Wilson et al., "Understanding Factors Influencing Vaccination Acceptance During Pregnancy Globally: A Literature Review," *Vaccine* 33, no. 47 (2015).

140   D. J. Jamieson and S. A. Rasmussen, "An Update on COVID-19 and Pregnancy," *American Journal of Obstetrics & Gynecology* 226, no. 2 (2022): 177.

141   Smriti Prasad et al., "Systematic Review and Meta-Analysis of the Effectiveness and Perinatal Outcomes of COVID-19 Vaccination in Pregnancy," *Nature Communications* 13, no. 1 (2022).

142   Tippi K. M. D. Mak et al., "Influenza Vaccination in Pregnancy: Current Evidence and Selected National Policies," *Lancet Infectious Diseases* 8, no. 1 (2008).

143   Ibid., 50; K. E. Wiley et al., "Pregnant Women's Intention to Take up a Post-Partum Pertussis Vaccine, and Their Willingness to Take up the Vaccine While Pregnant: A Cross Sectional Survey," *Vaccine* 31, no. 37 (2013); H. Blakeway et al., "COVID-19 Vaccination During Pregnancy: Coverage and Safety," *American Journal of Obstetrics & Gynecology* 226, no. 2 (2022).

144   Pranita D. M. D. Tamma et al., "Safety of Influenza Vaccination During Pregnancy," *American Journal of Obstetrics & Gynecology* 201, no. 6 (2009): 547.

145   Ibid., 548.

146   Male, "Are COVID-19 Vaccines Safe in Pregnancy?."; D. Di Mascio et al., "Outcome of Coronavirus Spectrum Infections (Sars, Mers, COVID-19) During Pregnancy: A systematic Systematic Review and Meta-Analysis," *American Journal of Obstetrics & Gynecology MFM* 2, no. 2 (2020).

147   Gayatri Amirthalingam et al., "Effectiveness of Maternal Pertussis Vaccination in England: An Observational Study," *Lancet* 384, no. 9953 (2014); K. Zaman et al., "Effectiveness of Maternal Influenza Immunization in Mothers and Infants," *The New England Journal of Medicine* 359, no. 15 (2008).

148   Heidi J. Larson, "Maternal Immunization: The New 'Normal' (or It Should Be)," *Vaccine* 33, no. 47 (2015): 6374.

149   WHO, "Weekly Epidemiological Record," (Global Advisory Committee on Vaccine Safety, 2013), 305.

150   Tamma et al., "Safety of Influenza Vaccination During Pregnancy," 548–50; Male, "Are COVID-19 Vaccines Safe in Pregnancy?"

151   WHO, "Weekly Epidemiological Record."

152   Sarah Geoghegan et al., "'This Choice Does Not Just Affect Me.' Attitudes of Pregnant Women toward COVID-19 Vaccines: A Mixed-Methods Study," *Human Vaccines & Immunotherapeutics* 17, no. 10 (2021).

153   David M. Oshinsky, *Polio: An American Story* (Oxford: Oxford University Press, 2005), 6; Duon H. Miller, "'Fake' Polio Vaccine May Kill Your Child," (Coral Gables, Florida: Polio Prevention Inc., 1956).

154   Gabrielle Calise, "Before the Coronavirus, Here's How Tampa Bay Fought Polio with Vaccines," *Tampa Bay Times*, https://www.tampabay.com/life-culture/history/2020/12/16/coronavirus-isnt-tampa-bays-first-vaccine-heres-

what-it-was-like-fighting-polio/; Nick Keppler, "The Loneliest Anti-Vaxxer," *Slate*, https://slate.com/news-and-politics/2021/11/polio-vaccine-antivaxxer-history-duon-miller.html.

155 Oshinsky, *Polio: An American Story*, 6.
156 Miller, "'Fake' Polio Vaccine May Kill Your Child." (his emphasis).

5 Starting strong
General guidelines for vaccine advocacy

Concern about vaccine hesitancy and misinformation is often joined by an interest in discovering what can be done in response. What, for example, are the most effective strategies for addressing vaccine doubts expressed by hesitant patients, close friends, or relatives? Regrettably, attempts to modify vaccine beliefs and behaviours provide the immediate lesson that changing people's views and actions around vaccination seems exceptionally difficult. Decades of research from across the globe that has investigated people's vaccine decision-making tendencies, attitudes, and behaviours has repeatedly concluded that trying to alter people's minds around immunisation can be unproductive. In fact, many interventions, including creative education-based efforts, seem to yield limited-or-no significant impacts, and increasing people's knowledge does not appear to substantially change vaccination-related beliefs and behaviours.[1] Bafflingly, while using carefully planned mass media campaigns can sometimes work, it seems that many intervention strategies may be disadvantageous and can even further entrench counter-vaccine beliefs.[2] At the same time, numerous approaches to tackling vaccine hesitancy are designed around limited amounts of empirical evidence to validate their use.[3] There is hope, however, and this chapter introduces key research-based methods, as well as five initial guidelines for improving vaccine advocacy.

The challenge of responding to vaccine hesitancy

Few effective, evidence-informed approaches to positively influencing people's vaccination attitudes and lessening opposition to vaccinations have been successfully identified. Sadly, it has been found that even doctors have resigned themselves to the futility of trying to sway vaccine hesitant parents, because they have experienced little success when attempting to change patients' vaccination beliefs and behaviours.[4] Ultimately, as the authors of an extensive study concluded, there is "no strong evidence on which to recommend any specific intervention to address vaccine hesitancy/refusal."[5] Although that news sounds disheartening, there are a handful of vaccine advocacy approaches that have demonstrated more promising results overall.

DOI: 10.4324/9781003312550-5

To start, researchers have tested various strategies for improving vaccine uptakes and have found that those categorised as behavioural intervention strategies, as well as efforts to deliver improved vaccination access, have met with the most success and empirical substantiation. Such interventions directly address the problem of access barriers that can often hinder people from getting vaccinated, and ways of positively influencing vaccination behaviours.

Behavioural strategies include providing monetary or nonmonetary incentives for vaccinating. This involves giving people some form of reward or acknowledgement for getting vaccinated. In association with incentives, it has been found that reducing logistical and economic barriers that obstruct individuals from getting vaccinated can be effective. The goal is simply to make vaccination easier. This might include subsidising people's travel expenses for getting vaccinated or reducing the cost of getting immunised through government subsidies, which might make vaccines free or comparatively inexpensive. If cost or time are barriers, then simply eliminating these obstacles can improve vaccine uptake. Along these lines, providing on-site vaccination drives at people's places of work can be very beneficial. If employees can get vaccinated with the annual flu shot at a place of work, during regular work hours, for instance, it makes it significantly easier for personnel to go ahead and get it. Correspondingly, many employers recognise that if they provide onsite vaccinations, and maintain a vaccinated workforce, it will be economically beneficially in the long term, because employees will be healthier and log fewer sick days. Alternative strategies include permitting allied health professionals, such as pharmacists and dentists, to administer an assortment of vaccines.[6] Individuals may find it easier to get vaccinated on a routine trip to the pharmacy, or while already at a dental appointment, than scheduling a separate visit to a GP.

Alternatively, the flipside to providing incentives involves imposing penalties for not vaccinating. In Australia, for instance, this approach has been embodied in the country's "No Jab No Pay" policy.[7] The policy removed conscientious objections on non-medical grounds from Australia's immunisation exemption criteria, and it limits government welfare assistance for families with low to middle incomes who have children not up to date on their immunisations. Under this scheme parents with children younger than 20 years of age, who are not fully vaccinated in line with the National Immunisation Program's schedule, are not eligible for state childcare payments and family tax rebates.

Another behavioural intervention strategy includes automatically setting people's vaccination appointments as the default option for individuals at their local medical clinic. A doctor's office may automatically schedule in vaccination appointments for patients, and then notify them of the upcoming date that they will need to attend. Such an approach is grounded within the notion of choice architecture, or *nudging*, which includes non-compulsory influences that do not necessarily restrict people's choices, but instead subtly alter the ways in which choices are presented. By making vaccination appointments the automatic, default condition for patients, the choice to opt-out of an automatically scheduled meeting is still available. However, the automatic setting of vaccine appointments, with opt-out choice construction, seems to lead people to take part more readily than if patients are required to choose to opt-in, and make the effort to schedule an appointment for themselves.

Along with analyses of behavioural interventions and improving access, numerous studies have identified that direct communications from health-care providers are frequently a key factor in increasing vaccination rates.[8] In fact, of all the determinants at play in vaccination choices, one of the strongest predictors of an individual's attitudes toward vaccines is whether a local family doctor delivered positive vaccine advocacy and advice in one-on-one appointment settings. People also seem likely to accept the opinion of the other healthcare and allied health professionals, including the advice of nurses and pharmacists, who are often highly respected and trusted, sometimes even more so than doctors.[9]

There are positives and negatives to each of these intervention techniques. For instance, imposing penalties for not vaccinating might backfire by eroding people's trust in the government and medical systems. Citizens might interpret such measures as attempts by policymakers to remove people's personal health choices and medical autonomy.[10] Also, policies such as Australia's No Jab No Pay legislation do not necessarily impact high income families, while they can disproportionately affect the poor. In terms of healthcare provider recommendations, it can also be logistically challenging, and even discouraging, for doctors to make regular efforts to answer the questions of vaccine doubting patients. Research has found that medical practitioners state that providing ongoing vaccine recommendations and answering questions for hesitant patients is not only time consuming, but it can lead to lower levels of job satisfaction.[11]

Additionally, many doctors and health workers who are in positions to provide direct, on-on-one interventions are not always doing so in the best possible ways. As researchers have found, clinicians engaging with vaccine hesitant patients often lack enhanced training in how to communicate using methods that are the most beneficial for bringing about vaccine acceptance.[12] In fact, studies have concluded that many science communicators require improved rhetoric, and increased awareness of media influences as they seek to challenge science-scepticism.[13] This includes learning how to use tools of persuasion rather than merely discussing scientific facts; because we know that vaccine decision-making is not only about knowledge or scientific literacy.[14]

Instead, healthcare practitioners can benefit from learning how to employ more convincing communication styles, since antivaccination messages are already actively using several persuasive cues. This is because, as the physician Douglas S. Diekema has suggested: "Data and facts, no matter how strongly supportive of vaccination, will not be sufficient to compete with the opposition's emotional appeals. The use of a compelling story about a single victim of vaccine-preventable illness is far more likely than data to move an audience to action."[15] In taking all this into account, it is necessary to take a deeper look at what pro-vaccination intervention strategies, communication approaches, and persuasion techniques researchers have benchmarked for improving vaccination uptakes.

Five general guidelines

Mike Klymkowsky has suggested that scientists "should stop trying to win arguments using the traditional academic approach, with data, error bars, and p-values, as these risk strengthening the emotional appeal of anti-evidence, anti-scientific viewpoints."[16] Instead, science advocates must consider how to "present data-based conclusions in compelling and effective ways, keeping in mind the connections and disconnections between human emotion and rationality." This is because people's decisions around matters of science "might have less to do with the message, and more about how – and in what context – the message is delivered." Klymkowsky's advice is a worthwhile starting point for those who want to improve vaccine advocacy. His words are a reminder to stop being focussed on trying to win arguments with facts and remember that the *ways* people communicate about vaccines can be just as important as the scientific data being presented.

In relation to this key advice, there are five general principles that should be considered for improving pro-vaccine advocacy:

1   Discard the Information Deficit Model
2   Be respectful, empathetic, and audience-focussed

    • Motivational Interviewing
    • The HURIER Model of Listening

3   Avoid verbal aggression
4   Be honest and open to questions
5   Acknowledge people's fears

These initial guidelines may appear simplistic, but they exemplify foundations upon which to start building better approaches to tackling vaccine hesitancy.

1 Discard the Information Deficit Model

From the outset, it is necessary to recall that the Information Deficit Model of science communication has been discredited (Chapter 2). Pro-vaccine advocacy must begin by accepting this reality. Remember that increasing people's factual knowledge and testable understanding of vaccines often does not translate into elevated levels of confidence in vaccination or improved immunisation behaviours.[17] Pro-vaccination advocates must admit that shortages of knowledge or public rationality are likely not a sufficient explanation for why vaccine hesitancy exists. As Seth Mnookin explained in his book, *The Panic Virus*, vaccine hesitant individuals he met were often well educated, and "took pride in being intellectually curious, thoughtful, and rational."[18]

Beyond people's knowledge of facts or theories are sociocultural beliefs and values. These are tied to community networks, and they frequently lied behind the public's vaccination attitudes. Consequently, merely conveying vaccine data will not necessarily make pro-vaccine communications effective. By contrast, trying to correct misinformation with accepted scientific facts can often be counterproductive, leading to reductions in people's intentions to vaccinate.[19] Even though communicating facts is important, better pro-vaccine advocacy needs to start by discarding the knowledge deficit myth.

2 Be respectful, empathetic and audience-focussed

Have you ever experienced poor customer service at a store or restaurant? Perhaps you have felt as though you have been treated with disrespect from an employee or a manager who has brushed off your complaints using an impolite tone or language. Such experiences can certainly be disconcerting. People can maintain long memories of the times when businesses have lacked empathy and failed to meet their expectations in terms of service quality or customer experience. In much the same way, individuals can be quick to remember negative interactions that they have had with medical professionals.

As noted in Chapter 2, past experiences can impact vaccine uptake. Disappointing encounters with healthcare workers or pro-vaccine messages can be pivotal in colouring perceptions against immunisation.[20] Therefore, it is essential to have positive interactions with vaccine hesitant individuals, and to produce constructive pro-vaccine messaging that is considerate of audiences. Though positive interactions may be time-costly, they start with respect, empathy, and striving to be audience-focussed. This advice is so vital that the Centres for Disease Control's best practices guidelines on immunisation recommend that physicians use empathetic communication with hesitant people.[21] Being respectful and audience-focussed includes dedicating time to listen to vaccine hesitant individuals and treating people with dignity. In fact, research has found that when medical professionals simply treat "each patient with respect and dignity" it increases the likelihood of patients following a doctor's advice.[22] With that in mind, it is also suggested that doctors never dismiss a family from their practice for vaccine refusal. This will not only be interpreted as discourteous, but it may hinder families from receiving quality health care, while ending future possibilities of communicating with patients about vaccines. It has also suggested that healthcare workers employ the audience-focussed dialogue technique of *Motivational Interviewing* (MI).

Motivational Interviewing

It might be tempting to simply dismiss people's vaccine doubts outright, because it is challenging to take time to thoughtfully respond to vaccine questions. However, interacting in a positive way, and being willing to respectfully listen, could play a decisive role in someone's vaccine decision-making processes while also building trust. Notably, one of the few vaccine hesitancy intervention strategies that has been found to result in compelling results involves using a conversation style known as Motivational Interviewing (MI). There is considerable evidence for the effectiveness of MI, and research has demonstrated its success in a variety of different settings.[23] So, what exactly is this intervention that is having success addressing vaccine hesitancy when many other techniques are not?

Motivational Interviewing is a person-centred method of dialogue that is intended to help change attitudes and behaviours by enhancing people's *own* internal motivations and resources.[24] As MI's founders have explained, "It involves guiding more than directing, dancing rather than wrestling, listening at least as much as telling."[25] MI is a conversation style that is more focussed on working with people than it is about just talking to them. It does this by exploring and getting to the bottom of people's ambivalence about change. Motivational Interviewing is intended to empathetically delve into an individual's concerns and reasons for change to address resistance against positive health behaviours. To do this, MI is grounded on the following characteristics, which are described as the "spirit" of Motivational Interviewing:[26]

A *Collaboration*. The intent is to form a relationship, and partner together on the decision-making process. This involves accepting every person at their own level of knowledge and being respectful of their views. The aim is to be empathetic and avoid arguing.

B *Evocation*. Through conversation, this consists of drawing out from people their own reasons and resources for change, which can include their own arguments, "personal goals, values, aspirations, and dreams."[27] MI then connects positive health decisions with the goals and values that people care about.

C *Honouring Autonomy*. This involves accepting people with empathy and acknowledging that they have their own autonomy to make choices.

Along with these characteristics are specific MI skills, which are consolidated in the acronym OARS (Open-ended questions, Affirmation, Reflecting, and Summary):[28]

1   *Open-ended questions.* These stand in contrast to closed questions, in which the answer is either *yes* or *no*. Instead, open-ended questions invite longer answers that encourage reflection. The goal is to allow the other individual to talk, rather than just talking at them. Such questions are intended to draw out a person's beliefs and ideas. Examples of such a question include the following:

- "I understand you have some concerns about the COVID-19 vaccines. Can you tell me about them?"[29]
- "Can you tell me what you've heard about [HPV or other] vaccines?"[30]
- "What do you think about the advantages of vaccination?"[31]

2   *Affirmation.* This involves acknowledging some positive characteristics about the individual, including their strengths, abilities, and pursuit of information. Affirmation promotes trust and builds confidence in the individual being interacted with. Illustrations may include:

- "You definitely care for your health, and I appreciate how much research you've done."
- "You have clearly been very resourceful coping with the difficulties during the COVID-19 pandemic."[32]

3   *Reflecting.* This consists of active listening, in which the listener offers a rephrased statement about what the individual has been being saying. Though reflecting may appear to be easy, it takes effort to do well. It is done to better understand the person's perceptions while restating their feelings and viewpoints for clarity.

- "I get where you're coming from. It sounds like you're saying that it's confusing how there is a great deal of conflicting COVID-19 vaccination information out there, and you don't know who to trust."[33]
- "As you said, vaccines have reduced diseases in such an important way that they are now much less frequent. It's why you have vaccinated your child when he was a baby. If I understood you correctly, with the exception of measles vaccine, other vaccines seem safe to you."[34]

4   *Summary.* This is a special use of the reflection skill that is often applied near the end of a conversation, or utilised to link ideas together. Summaries are employed to ensure that there is clear communication taking place between conversation participants, and to demonstrate that you have been listening. They can also prompt an individual to elaborate further. Here are examples of such summaries:

- "So you are saying that if you get vaccinated you fear you might experience an allergic reaction similar to the ones you experienced as a result of eating peanuts."[35]

- "So, you find that it's important to protect your child against diseases when the vaccines are safe, but you're worried about what you've heard regarding autism and [the] measles vaccine."[36]

The HURIER Model of Listening

At the heart of Motivational Interviewing's OARS is respectful listening and empathetic dialogue. When MI is applied to vaccine hesitancy, this means paying close attention to an individual's questions about vaccines and attempting to restate a person's concerns to ensure that their misgivings are fully understood. It also means trying to see things from the perspective of a vaccine hesitant individual. Importantly, listening itself is a competency that can be sharpened with practice. One method of improving listening aptitude for the purposes of Motivational Listening and positive dialogue includes the HURIER model of listening. This model is a practical framework for understanding and enhancing listening abilities.

A clear challenge of MI is that it takes time and sincere listening. Our daily lives are often filled with numerous distractions, as we make our way in a world of connected technologies, social networks, multitasking, and other demands on our attention. Our phones are sending us notifications from the time that we wake up until when we go to bed. Emails, calendar notifications, and media alerts seem to always be diverting our attention while we are trying to complete work tasks and attempt to listen to colleagues, students, family members, customers, or patients. With all these potential diversions chiming away, you may have experienced being in a conversation with someone who was noticeably giving sidelong glances to their phones while you are attempting to interact with them. It can give you the feeling that the other person might be hearing you, but not truly listening. Such scenarios can be frustrating. In this modern atmosphere of steady interruptions, being heard, and really listening to others can sometimes seem more uncommon than they ought to be.

It also appears as there can be a concerted focus in professional development training on improving leaders' speaking skills to others and investing in becoming better communicators to audiences. Yet there can be a noticeable lack of emphasis on improving listening abilities in our workplaces and professional operations. As it turns out, being able to listen, and listening well, is a crucial skill that can make or break interactions with vaccine hesitant individuals. It is also a skill that can be learned for Motivational Interviewing purposes. Listening is a craft that can be refined, and by cultivating your listening abilities, you can create opportunities for enhanced dialogue with hesitant people.

The HURIER model of listening was developed by Professor Judi Brownell to improve listening competencies. It is a simplified, skills-based framework for listening, which includes six interrelated components.[37] HURIER is the acronym for these six components, or skill areas, which

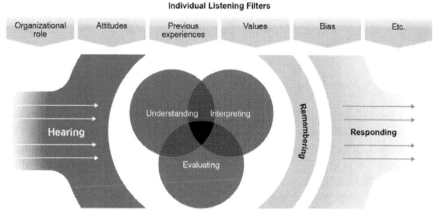

Figure 5.1 The Six-Component HURIER Listening Process[41]

include the following steps of the listening process: *Hearing, Understanding, Remembering, Interpreting, Evaluating,* and *Responding.* Hearing, of course, is an important part of good listening, and it is the "prerequisite to all listening that involves vocal communication, regardless of the purpose."[38] According to Brownell, hearing simply involves the "accurate reception of sounds."[39] This is the mechanical process of taking in sounds, and for most of us hearing occurs all the time as a constant physiological process. But to really hear someone competently, you "must focus your attention, discriminate among sounds, and concentrate."[40]

Astute hearing requires the deliberate reduction of distractions and interruptions, while trying to maintain mental attentiveness to the verbal, as well as nonverbal messages that someone is trying to communicate.[42] Hearing is influenced not only by external factors, such as distractions, but by internal factors, including our attitudes, biases, past experiences, our interests, values, and worldviews, which can act as filters to what we are really hearing or choosing not to hear.[43] We may be prone to filtering out messages that we do not want to listen to, or not really hearing certain people at all. The listening skill of truly hearing, therefore, requires concentration, it takes energy, and it can be improved as a skill.

Understanding is the comprehension component of listening. It goes beyond hearing and involves recognising and making sense of the words or symbols being communicated and computing the meaning of what has been heard.[44] One way to ensure understanding is to ask questions, when it is appropriate without interrupting, to clarify that you grasp what someone is actually trying to communicate.[45] Another procedure for improving understanding is simply listening to someone's entire message, without cutting in on them. Brownell has noted, "The urge to interrupt is the greatest when you have strong opinions and are listening to someone who also appears certain of his viewpoint." Also, sometimes longwinded communicators need to be interrupted to allow for the free flow of ideas.[46] However, understanding can often be improved by limiting interruptions.

Remembering incorporates the recall systems involved in storing and acting upon what has been heard and understood in the listening process. Memory allows us to capture what is being communicated, and then respond in due process. Remembering is the component of listening that allows us to "act on what is received, either immediately or at some later point in time," and it provides the "ability to formulate an appropriate response."[47] One strategy for improving memory while listening involves trying to engage your visual memory system while listening.[48] Using your imagination, try to visualise in your mind's eye what the person you are listening to is trying to communicate as vividly and creatively as possible.

Interpreting involves taking "into account the total communication context so that you are better able to understand the meaning of what is said from the speaker's point of view."[49] This involves trying to empathise with the speaker's own perspective, to not simply understand, but to also understand the message from the other person's perspective. Accurate interpretation requires that you observe nonverbal cues. To improve interpreting, you should try to pay active attention to a communicator's facial expressions, posture, and hand gestures, while also letting someone know that they have been understood. Interpreting is really the relational and empathetic component of listening, and it involves social sensitivities and trying to hear "what is *not* said."[50]

Evaluating is "the process by which an individual makes a judgment about the accuracy and validity of the information received."[51] The issue with evaluating is that it should not be concluded too hastily. Instead, effective evaluating "requires withholding evaluation until a message has been completely understood."[52] First-rate listening involves making sure that you "have complete and accurate information before making a decision," and trying to be aware of one's own biases and values that can influence your objectivity.[53] Evaluating should incorporate "critical listening," which involves thoughtfully weighing every aspect of what is being communicated. This means evaluating all parts of a message, including its purpose, the credibility of the speaker, and whether the communication contains persuasive cues.[54]

Responding is the outcome of listening, and it should be informed by the previous five components.[55] It is still embedded in the listening process, because excellent responding occurs in the context of Hearing, Understanding, Remembering, Interpreting, and Evaluating. Responding delivers your feedback to the communicator, which incorporates verbal, spoken components, but also nonverbal aspects of a response, including hand gestures and facial expressions. What is important about the HURIER model, and becoming a better listener, is that the responding component is conceptualised as only one-sixth of the whole listening process. In this regard, effective communication involves all six components of the listening process, not merely speaking. People will "judge the effectiveness of your listening by the nature of the response you make to what you hear."[56] Consequently, what is vital to consider for better responding is engaging in the five other components of listening before you speak.

In the end, if you want to enhance one-one-on interactions with vaccine hesitant individuals, you should seek to become a better listener in the context of Motivational Interviewing. Effective listening can be achieved by focussing on the six components of the HURIER model and trying to improve on each skill area as you interact with the people around you. This is because, "Effective communication begins with effective listening," and, "Unless you listen well, you cannot hope to communicate effectively."[57]

3 Avoid verbal aggression

When communicating with vaccine hesitant individuals it is essential to avoid verbal aggression. Verbal aggressiveness includes ridicule and attacks on people's character, competence, or ridiculing someone's background or appearance.[58] There is little to be gained from such adversarial styles of communicating, because aggressive language is unlikely to sway vaccine hesitant audiences. Ridiculing people's sources of counter-vaccine information is also unhelpful.[59] In the same vein, trying to shame or frighten vaccine hesitant patients can be counterproductive.[60]

Even though antivaccination messages are factually untrue, and you may feel very strongly about the benefits of vaccinating, it is still important to refrain from being hostile. Aggressive language can be polarising, and people react negatively to being ridiculed or treated as unintelligent. Research has also found that verbal aggression decreases an audience's perceptions of a communicator's credibility in both offline and online environments.[61] Additionally, verbal aggression may lower people's interest in a message, it can reduce an audience's motivation to learn, and it can decrease a communicator's likeability.[62] Though health workers can be assertive about the safety and effectiveness of vaccines, it is disadvantageous to be verbally uncivil to vaccine hesitant individuals.

4 Be honest and open to questions

In Chapter 2 it was noted that scepticism toward doctors and healthcare authorities, and distrust of the government can impact on vaccination uptake.[63] People also frequently express a lack of trust in pharmaceutical companies and health systems, while they can be sceptical of pro-vaccine information. This is why pro-vaccine advocates need to be honest and open to questions, because any hint of dishonesty or intolerance of queries will stoke pre-existing scepticism. Honesty is also part and parcel of being respectful, which means being candid about vaccination side effects.

Additionally, being honest necessitates communicating to hesitant individuals that vaccines represent one of the most significant breakthroughs in medical history, and they save countless lives while delivering important community benefits. Candour also entails being truthful about the potential for serious illnesses that may result from vaccine preventable diseases, which makes failing to vaccinate a risky prospect.

5 Acknowledge people's fears

Fear can be a powerful motivator. In fact, as identified in Chapter 2, vaccine fears and risk calculations are notable factors that can lessen people's likelihood of getting vaccinated. Importantly, such fears may be associated with people's desire to protect their family and to keep children safe from potential harm. Even though fears about vaccine safety may not be scientifically valid, they can stem from genuine concern for the wellbeing of loved ones. It is necessary, therefore, to accept that parents who "refuse vaccination are not acting frivolously or recklessly."[64] Instead, they likely "just want what is best for their children, even if in this case, based on current scientific evidence, they are mistaken." Consequently, such anxieties should not simply be dismissed, because worries about child safety are deep seated and part of the everyday experience of being a parent. As a result, brushing off people's safety concerns could be perceived as devaluing people's gut feelings about safeguarding the people they love.

Dismissing people's vaccine qualms can also provoke distrust. As Jennifer A. Reich has stated, "Although much data suggest that parents dramatically overestimate the risks of vaccines, many providers and public health groups might be too eager to dismiss these risks and shortcomings for fear of encouraging parents to opt out." Unfortunately, this tendency may be causing health professionals to "lose the ability to discuss these uncertainties, which, in turn, fuels distrust of authority and a broader misunderstanding of science."[65] Instead, it is important to acknowledge a questioning person's fears, and to affirm that their desire to safeguard the health of their family is a positive impulse. This connects with people's emotional sensitivities rather than discounting them, and it opens the door to further discussions. As Claire Hooker has explained: "A fearful parent needs to know we care about their concerns on say, vaccine safety, and that we have heard and understood their worries. That's before they will care about what we say."[66]

The need for improved vaccine advocacy

Ultimately, pro-vaccine advocacy ought to be built around respect and audience-focus. This means putting yourself into the shoes of vaccine doubters and empathising with hesitant individuals rather than attacking them. It should also involve being honest and open to questions and acknowledging people's fears. Taking into account such advice, pro-vaccine advocacy can likely be improved on a number of fronts. Certainly, researchers have concluded that counter-vaccination media outperforms pro-vaccine efforts in terms of the sheer number of websites and social media posts that antivaccinationists produce, as well as in regard to the apparent persuasiveness of such online messages.[67] Studies have also concluded that science advocates, such as vaccine supporters, have time and again failed to address numerous counter-scientific claims in compelling ways that might appeal to audiences.[68] Antivaccination messages are more abundant and they may be more persuasive than pro-vaccination media.

As a result, there is a glaring demand for improved vaccination advocacy, and better training is needed regarding how to effectively address people's immunisation concerns.[69] Improving pro-vaccine advocacy involves taking into account tools of rhetoric and learning about persuasive cues. It also requires learning about the nuances of how people are persuaded and make decisions, as well as acknowledging the influences of media and counter-vaccine messages.[70] All in all, pro-vaccine advocacy can likely be improved on a number of fronts to rival the remarkably widespread, persuasive, and psychologically sticky nature of antivaccination messages. On that account, the remainder of this chapter will supplement the five general guidelines for vaccine advocacy by also examining behaviour-modification techniques, as well as the importance of healthcare provider interactions. This will be followed with suggestions on how to address cultural cognition, the value of affirming people's autonomy of choice, and need to be mindful of biases.

Behaviour-modification techniques

When considering how to potentially modify vaccination behaviours, it must be reiterated that a key factor in low vaccine uptakes is access barriers.[71] Remember that access barriers consist of logistical and scheduling difficulties, lack of time, and the financial costs of getting vaccinated, which can make getting vaccinated a difficult option for some people.[72] As a result, if you are concerned about increasing vaccination rates, a useful starting point to help swiftly boost community uptake is to identify ways of removing such barriers. Policymakers, civic leaders, and health workers should consider what possibilities are available for making vaccination less costly and more convenient. In addition to improving access, researchers have also found that among the many strategies that have been trialled for improving vaccination rates, those which have met with the greatest success involve specific behavioural intervention techniques and choice architecture. These interventions include providing monetary and nonmonetary incentives, imposing penalties for not vaccinating, and tailoring how vaccination options are framed as well as using nudges.

Incentives and penalties

The appeal of offering incentives seems obvious, and research has indicated that cash incentives can improve health behaviours and potentially influence vaccination uptake.[73] However, the use of incentives can have mixed results and they may not necessarily be cost-effective. They can also be more appealing to individuals in lower economic brackets than to high-income households.[74] Alternatively, imposing penalties can also increase vaccination rates. In the years following Australia's enactment of its penalty-based No Jab No Pay policy, for instance, hundreds of thousands of children were brought up to date with the national immunisation schedule. However, imposing penalties can also backfire by generating psychological reactance. As one study concluded, "Overall it is felt that *No Jab, No Pay* has had little effect on the views of those who object to the concept of vaccination, except to reinforce their negativity around the subject, as they now feel the government is "forcing" people to vaccinate their children."[75]

Choice architecture and nudging

In contrast with incentives or penalties are the related concepts of choice architecture and nudging. Choice architecture has been described as interventions that "involve altering the properties or placement of objects or stimuli within micro-environments with the intention of changing health-related behaviour."[76] These can include "changing the size of plates, bowls or glasses, or placing less healthy foods further away from customers in a cafeteria" to encourage healthier eating behaviours.[77] Correspondingly, Richard H. Thaler and Cass R. Sunstein have explained that a nudge is "any aspect of the choice architecture that alters people's behaviour in a predictable way without forbidding any options or significantly changing their economic incentives."[78] As they clarify, "To count as a mere nudge, the intervention must be easy and cheap to avoid. Nudges are not mandates. Putting the fruit at eye level counts as a nudge. Banning junk food does not."

Choice architecture in action includes automatically enrolling employees into a retirement savings plan, rather than requiring them to sign on to such a scheme. This nudges people to save more for retirement. One of the most famous illustrations of successful nudging is the urinal fly:

> A wonderful example of this principle comes from, of all places, the men's rooms at Schiphol Airport in Amsterdam. There the authorities have etched the image of a black housefly into each urinal. It seems that men usually do not pay much attention to where they aim, which can create a bit of a mess, but if they see a target, attention and therefore accuracy are much increased. According to the man who came up with the idea, it works wonders. "It improves the aim," says Aad

Kieboom. "If a man sees a fly, he aims at it." Kieboom, an economist, directs Schiphol's building expansion. His staff conducted fly-in-urinal trials and found that etchings reduce spillage by 80 percent.[79]

With the urinal fly nudge, people are neither rewarded nor punished for their (in-)accuracy. Men are not forced to aim at the fly, yet the presence of such a target nudges people to take better aim.

A nudge that has been used to increase vaccination rates involves making routine childhood vaccination appointments the default option for patients. With this nudge, a physician's office automatically schedules required vaccination appointments for the practice's patients, so that individuals must actively opt-out if they do not want themselves or their family members vaccinated.[80] Through such choice architecture, vaccination remains non-compulsory, but the decision-making environment is configured so that the patient must voluntarily decline the appointment. This type of opt-out choice construction may increase vaccination receipt, in contrast with opt-in designs that require patients to make immunisation appointments for themselves.[81]

The importance of healthcare provider interactions

Despite people's scepticism and distrust of experts, healthcare professionals are still highly respected sources of vaccine information.[82] Vaccination recommendations from doctors, nurses, and pharmacists can be one of the most influential factors in vaccine decision-making, and people's experiences with health workers can directly impact whether people choose to accept or reject vaccinations.[83] Vaccine information and assurances about vaccine safety provided by health providers in one-on-one appointments *does* change people's minds about vaccination.[84] This is especially the case when such interactions employ Motivational Interviewing (see p. 135).

However, the influence of health workers is not always positive. In fact, negative experiences with health providers, and poor communication by medical professionals about vaccines, are key reasons why people decline or delay vaccination.[85] This is why it is essential that medical practitioners adopt the five general guidelines for improved pro-vaccine advocacy discussed above. Additionally, more specific techniques of communication and styles of patient engagement can be utilised by healthcare professionals to positively influence immunisation behaviours. These include employing the following strategies:

1   Presumptive announcements
2   Social Consensus
3   Future intentions and self-predictive questions
4   Telling stories
5   Reminders

1 Presumptive announcements

It has been found that vaccine acceptance increases when doctors frame the option of getting vaccinated in presumptive announcements, which highlight how vaccination is the norm and the assumed default action for all patients.[86] Instead of listing options, and the choice of *not* getting vaccinated, clinicians can experience better outcomes when they simply make it known that a patient is due for a vaccine and needs to receive it as soon as is possible. This can involve stating that the individual or family member will be receiving the required shot today in accordance with national guidelines, or, that they will now be scheduled in for an appointment as is routine for all patients.[87] In effect, this communication approach utilises choice architecture in that such presumed statements present an opt-out, rather than an opt-in scenario. So, stating presumptively that, "Your child needs to be vaccinated today," or, "We will book in an appointment now for the vaccinations your child needs," will be more effective than remarking, "You should consider having your child vaccinated."

2 Social Consensus

It may also be valuable to communicate in ways that utilise Social Consensus. Chapter 3 considered Social Consensus in relation to the Confidence theme of antivaccination media. This same persuasive cue, and in particular social proof messaging, can also enhance healthcare worker consultations. Social proof involves referring to the beliefs and behaviours of others and emphasising that many people agree with an idea, or action, or use a certain product. Hence, a healthcare professional may add a social proof declaration to a presumptive announcement. In such cases it may be stated that a patient will be receiving a vaccine today. A medical worker can then add that the vaccine is routine for all of the other patients attending the practice, and that it is accepted by the majority of people according to the national immunisation schedule.[88]

Employing Social Consensus is important because many people choose to get vaccinated because they believe that the majority of people are also doing so.[89] Researchers of vaccine uptake have noted that there exists "considerable evidence that letting people know what other people do is one of the most effective ways of increasing that behavior."[90] Relatedly, it has been found that individuals tend be more open to immunisation when getting vaccinated is described as a social norm. Consequently, health works should use presumptive announcements that reference the participating majority of people who are also joining in on the default, prescriptive action of getting vaccinated.

When mentioning that vaccination is a social norm, it can also be helpful to point out that vaccines are a *social good*. Remind patients that getting vaccinated is a beneficial act that aids the whole community. People's

vaccination choices have important consequences for others, and not vaccinating may risk spreading a preventable disease to family members, friends,
and people in the wider community who may not be able to get vaccinated. Refusing or delaying vaccination could endanger infants, pregnant
friends, elderly relatives, or immunocompromised cancer patients and organ
transplant recipients.[91]

3 Future intentions and self-predictive questions

Chapter 4 touched upon the persuasive cue described as Asking Questions
in the Danger theme of antivaccination media. Medical workers can also
employ questions about a patient's future intentions to improve one-on-one
appointments. Williams, Fitzsimmons, and Block have explained that
answering a "seemingly innocuous question regarding future intentions" can
significantly persuade an audience's behaviour towards those same intentions.[92] For instance, if individuals are simply asked to make predictions
about their anticipated actions, such as whether they would be willing to
predict how much time they may spend volunteering for a local charity,
they are appreciably more likely to initially overcommit to, and then later
carry out, that behaviour. Answering intention questions can cause "automatic or nonconscious changes in cognitive structure that lead to behavioural changes of which the respondent is often not aware."[93] Accordingly,
prompting patients to consider their future intentions to vaccinate, and
encouraging clients to formulate date-specific plans to fulfil these immunisation targets, has demonstrated positive results.[94]

4 Telling stories

As highlighted in Chapter 4, antivaccination media are steeped in emotionally charged personal stories about vaccination dangers.[95] Though such
antivaccine narratives are factually dubious, stories have proven to be influential communication tools that may trigger peripheral route processing,
and appear to be more persuasive than systematic, well-reasoned arguments.[96] That point must be reiterated: *stories are often more persuasive than
logical, fact-centred arguments* (Chapter 6).[97] Stories also seem to transcend
education levels, they can give rise to influential emotional reactions, and
they can generate empathy because people often personally self-identify
with a storyline's characters, contexts and the values that might be communicated through a good narrative.[98]

At the same time, *narrative-framing*, which involves positioning information within culturally sympathetic narratives, has been proposed as a means
for reducing culturally cognitive reactance to scientific ideas.[99] As a result,
researchers strongly suggest that vaccine advocates share narratives about
people suffering from vaccine-preventable diseases, or personal anecdotes
about how someone chose to get one's own family members vaccinated.[100]

Tell stories about how you or others became convinced of vaccine safety and effectiveness, and work at becoming a better storyteller. This is vital because antivaccinationists have long been recounting their own anecdotes about vaccines and their supposed dangers, which can be cognitively sticky even if they are based on misinformation.

The power of hearing personal experiences with vaccine-preventable diseases was demonstrated in a 2019 study titled, "Combating Vaccine Hesitancy with Vaccine-Preventable Disease Familiarization."[101] The study incorporated 574 college students. 491 of these students were identified as pro-vaccine and 83 were categorised as vaccine hesitant. Approximately half of the students were put into a treatment group, and they were tasked with interviewing a family or community member who had experienced a vaccine-preventable disease. The other half were assigned to the control group, which involved interviewing someone with an auto-immune disease. The treatment group heard stories from people who had personal experience with a vaccine-preventable disease, and the pain and suffering that such illnesses can cause:

> One student interviewed a member of their church congregation who had shingles: "The pain was so bad that she ended up at a pain management clinic where they did steroid shots into her spine. The pain meds didn't even touch [reduce] her pain, even the heavy ones. For months she couldn't leave the house." This interview led the student to explain...that "The project showed how the lack of vaccination is essentially accepting the pain and suffering that comes with disease." Another student interviewed his or her grandmother about tuberculosis: "Before getting diagnosed and during the time that she was treated, she could work her eight-hour temple shift and then she would go straight to bed after getting home. After a couple of hours nap, she would get up for a short time to get small tasks done before retiring to bed for the night." This student summarized the interview experience as "I dislike the idea of physical suffering so hearing about someone getting a disease made the idea of getting a disease if I don't get vaccinated seem more real."[102]

In the end, 68% of the students in the intervention group who had been classified as vaccine hesitant became pro-vaccine. Exposure to firsthand accounts of the real-world impacts of vaccine-preventable disease, therefore, can "significantly improve attitudes towards vaccination."[103]

5 Reminders

One of the most reliable indicators of people's attitudes toward vaccines is whether their local health workers delivered positive vaccine advocacy and advice in one-on-one appointment settings. However, it might be challenging to get patients in the door for such helpful one-on-one appointments and consultations in the first place. To overcome this problem, studies indicate that primary healthcare providers should send vaccination reminders to clients. Delivering postcards and update letters, texting, or phoning patients to remind people of their vaccine needs positively impacts immunisation rates.[104] Such reminders increase people's exposure to vaccine requirements beyond clinical settings, and they boost memory recall of immunisation needs that they may have otherwise not thought about in everyday life.

Address Cultural Cognition

At the heart of research-informed advice about how to improve pro-vaccine advocacy is an overarching need to be audience-focussed first. Audience-focussed science advocacy involves more than just concentrating on communicating facts. It means empathising with vaccine hesitant individuals and being respectful rather than trying to win arguments. In considering what it means to be audience-focussed, it is vital to be mindful the Cultural Cognition Thesis, and the effects of identity-protective cognition (Chapter 2). Remember that the Cultural Cognition Thesis maintains that individuals can reject scientific consensus on such matters as climate change and vaccines, not simply because they lack information about these topics. Instead, people tend to accept whatever position reinforces their connection to other people with whom they share significant social and cultural ties.[105] Those who reject the safety and effectiveness of vaccines are often aware of the scientific consensus on vaccination, and their rejection of vaccines is not necessarily associated with low scientific literacy or even a lack of knowledge. According to identity-protective cognition, people selectively accept or deny scientific facts in ways that reflect what they already believe, in relation to the worldviews maintained by the cultural groups that they self-identify with.[106]

Correspondingly, people tend to use a type of social-cultural logic to sift through scientific facts and theories, and they are likely to reject ideas, and expert advice, that contradict their own cultural identities. These identities are linked to the viewpoints accepted by the groups that individuals are personally connected with. For this reason, learning more facts does not inevitably change minds, especially if those facts seem to conflict with the cultural values and beliefs held by the people with whom social ties are closely held. Plus, if vaccine misinformation supports someone's central worldview, it is more likely to be accepted than scientific data. Trying to correct that vaccine misinformation with factual claims can then be interpreted as an attack on one's core beliefs.[107] As Dan Kahan has concluded, "The practical lesson, then, is pretty clear. Don't simply bombard people with information." In fact, trying to do that "can actually provoke a cultural identity-protective backlash" which may make people less likely to accept the scientific data.[108] Identity-protective cognition is an identity self-defence mechanism, that kicks in to try to shield our social and cultural values against perceived threats from experts and scientific facts.[109]

If vaccine supporters truly want to be audience-focussed, therefore, it is essential to launch pro-vaccine advocacy by thinking first about cultural cognition, identity-protection, and an audience's worldviews. Bearing that in mind, there are two cultural cognition game plans that should be considered in order to develop better audience-focussed advocacy. The first involves using *cultural-identity affirmation*. This involves trying to present scientific facts in ways that affirm people's cultural identities, rather than threatening them.[110] For example, in one experiment Dan Kahan's research team had two groups of subjects read a newspaper article that reported about a "study issued by a panel of scientists from major universities who found definitive evidence that the temperature of the earth is increasing." The study indicated that the temperature increase was human caused, and that "the consequences of continued global warming would be catastrophic for the environment and the economy." In the experiment, one research groups had been told that the "the study had called for the institution of stronger antipollution controls." These controls would feature government policies and corporate restrictions that would likely threaten the identity of hierarchical-individualists. These are people who score toward the top of the Grid scale, in the direction of Hierarchy, and those who would score toward the left of the Group scale, on the side of Individualism, in relation to the Cultural Cognition Map (Figure 5.2).

Bear in mind that hierarchical-individualists tend to value free enterprise and business success, and they often contend that governments should not overregulate society. Such persons are inclined to be the most sceptical of

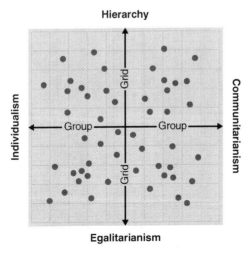

Figure 5.2 Cultural Cognition Map[111]

climate change science, because it brings with it the need for environmental guidelines for corporations that may hinder commerce.[112] For the other group in the experiment, however, the article was altered to state that the panel of scientists recommended a "removal on restrictions on nuclear power, so that American society could substitute nuclear power for greenhouse gas emitting fossil fuel energy sources."[113] Hierarchical-individualists are not threatened by the idea of nuclear power, and that version of the experiment called for less government restrictions on nuclear energy production, which would be in line with individualistic values that call out for fewer government regulations.

In both of the experiment's scenarios, the panel of scientists reported on empirical data about the earth becoming warmer because of human caused influences. Yet both proposed different solutions, with one calling for more antipollution regulations, and the other recommending fewer regulations of some variety. What Kahan's team found was that hierarchical-individualists were significantly more likely to accept the same scientific findings when they read the article that called for a removal of restrictions, because that solution affirmed the audience's core cultural identities. It was also discovered that hierarchical-individualists "who received the newspaper report that recommended antipollution controls were even more skeptical of the reported factual findings of the study" than were hierarchical-individualists in "a control group who received no newspaper story on the findings of the scientists."[114] When the exact same science was interpreted as threatening hierarchical-individualist values it was more resisted, and the facts backfired because of identity-protective cognition. As Dan Kahan concluded, we should not "try to convince people to accept a solution by showing them there is a problem." Instead, "Show them a solution they find culturally affirming, and then they are disposed to believe there really is a problem in need of solving."[115]

The second cultural cognition game plan for better audience-focussed pro-vaccine advocacy involves using *pluralistic advocacy*. Remember that people are more likely to trust an expert, and the facts that they communicate, if the expert shares the same worldview of the audience. "People feel that it is safe to consider evidence with an open mind when they know that a knowledgeable member of their cultural community accepts it."[116] However, individuals also tend to judge experts to be untrustworthy if the specialist seems to be opposed to their own cultural values. In response to such inclinations, it has been suggested that cultural-cognitive polarisation can be reduced by using pluralistic advocacy.[117] This involves purposefully featuring several experts who represent numerous worldviews and cultural outlooks. When a diverse set of experts, from a range of sociocultural backgrounds, together advocate for the same science, the diversity neutralises feelings that the science is linked with a single worldview.[118] When pluralistic advocacy is employed, individuals may still disagree about the scientific facts, but "they are less likely to do so along strictly cultural lines," and they will be more inclined to consider "information in an open-minded way."[119] It has even been suggested that "the impact of cultural cognition would be relatively small if citizens observed persons of diverse values on both sides of the mandatory vaccination debate."[120]

Being audience-focussed brings with it the need to accept that science "information must be transmitted in a form that makes individuals' acceptance of it compatible with their core cultural commitments."[121] It is simply not enough "that the information be true; it must be framed in a manner that bears an acceptable social meaning" through cultural-identity affirmation. Additionally, identity-protective self-defence can be mitigated by delivering information through pluralistic advocacy in order to foster open-mindedness.

Affirm autonomy of choice

Chapter 2 introduced the idea of psychological reactance, which may be a key factor in vaccine decision-making. This is because mandatory vaccination policies can be interpreted as forceful restrictions of medical choices and civic freedoms.[122] It is worthwhile, therefore, to take psychological reactance into account when interacting with vaccine hesitant individuals. Remember that people can reflexively oppose losing their freedoms of behaviour and can reject authoritative commands to vaccinate if such orders are perceived to be coercive.[123] Consequently, it is of value to affirm people's autonomy of choice around vaccination, and to reinforce that in the end they have the freedom to make important immunisation decisions.[124]

Verbally respecting people's autonomy can be important for opening up further conversations, and health workers can empower hesitant individuals by asking them whether they would like more information on vaccines to make their own informed decisions.[125] It is vital that medical professionals directly communicate about the safety and efficacy of vaccines, as well as the risks associated with not vaccinating, yet still acknowledge that patients have their own decision-making rights. Affirming people's right to choose is an act of respect, which may also defuse feelings of reactance and trigger profitable conversations.

Be mindful of biases

Judi Brownell's HURIER model of listening touches upon the roles that biases can play in the listening process. Brownell explains that biases can impact the Hearing component by influencing what messages are listened to, and which ones might be filtered out.[126] Additionally, successful Evaluating necessitates that a listener is aware of his or her own biases, because biases can skew our judgements about the accuracy and legitimacy of the information being listened to. Such basic observations point to the fact that there is value in being mindful of our own biases, as well as the potential biases of those with whom we are trying to communicate.

The word bias means to have a "one-sided tendency or direction" and to be inclined "to one side," perhaps unfairly so.[127] Not all biases are necessarily problematic, because some may reflect more accurate perceptions of the world. For instance, maintaining a bias toward accepting data found in peer-reviewed research, produced by trained scientific experts, over-and-against information from non-academic social media posts can be quite beneficial. Such a partiality may not lead to perfect results, but even that preference is still a bias. Whether they are beneficial or not, every person has social and political biases that are shaped by our upbringing, education, and experiences. These biases can be culturally cognitive, and they colour our views of experts and academic research, even though we are not overtly conscious of them. In fact, if one thinks that they do not have any biases, that opinion is likely a biased misperception about themselves connected with low intellectual humility (Chapter 2).

When communicating with vaccine hesitant individuals, it is important to be mindful of our own biases, while also keeping in mind the potential biases of people with vaccination doubts.[128] It is helpful to be aware of subtle psychological biases that can often influence the ways that people process information and impact vaccine decision-making. These include the *Confirmation bias*, the *Omission bias*, the *Availability heuristic*, the *Negativity bias*, and the *Narrative bias*. Regarding the first of these, the Confirmation bias is a tendency to seek out and favour facts that fit our pre-existent beliefs. We tend to only look for evidence that confirms what we already think is true, and we are disposed to ignore or trivialise evidence that disconfirms our existing beliefs.[129] If parents already believe that vaccines are dangerous, for instance, they will be less likely to accept facts that refute the belief and will be biased toward stories and information that confirm it.

The Omission bias relates to a psychological preference toward harm caused by inaction rather than harm resulting from our own choices. This is because we tend to feel moral culpability for harm that comes from our actions, which seems worse than harm that might result from not acting.[130] Parents may prefer, therefore, not to have their children vaccinated because acting, and choosing to have their kids immunised, would mean that any theoretical harm resulting from the vaccine would fall onto their own shoulders.[131] For example, in one study "participants were presented with a [hypothetical] scenario in which a child faces a 10 in 10,000 risk of dying from the flu." They were told that a "vaccine eliminates this risk but can itself cause the flu in rare cases, resulting in a 5 in 10,000 risk of death from the vaccine." The experiment's vaccine option represents a significant decrease in risk. Many participants still chose to refuse the vaccine, however, which indicated that they thought that "death from the disease is more acceptable than a death from the vaccine (even if it is more likely)."[132] Participating individuals supposed that by having their children vaccinated they would feel more responsible because of their decision to act, than if their child died as a result of not vaccinating.

The Availability heuristic is a mental shortcut that leads us to draw conclusions quickly based upon what comes immediately to our minds. This means that when we make decisions, we often give more weight to ideas that are the most readily accessible to us in our memories. Interestingly, what our memory frequently recalls can often be rare but noteworthy events, because they are more emotionally striking or unique, making them psychologically gripping. For example, people can judge air travel to be far more dangerous than driving in a car, because the rare plane crashes that are reported in media are more memorable. Newscasts about much scarcer airplane disasters, therefore, might spring to mind faster than the many more common car accidents we hear about on a day-to-day basis. We then misjudge air travel to be more hazardous, even though it is statistically a much safer mode of transport. The same tendency can be at play in vaccination decision-making.[133] For instance, "A vividly portrayed narrative about a child who had a bad vaccine reaction can cause parents to overestimate the probability of their own child having a reaction," since emotionally arresting stories can stand out in our memories.[134]

The Negativity bias is a common tendency to give more weight to negative information. It is also part-and-parcel of the Contrast Principle and Negativity Effect discussed in Chapter 4. With this bias people tend to trust data, and have more confidence in studies, which report that there are possible health risks associated with a potential hazard. They do this over and against positive studies indicating that there is no need to be worried about possible health risks associated with a prospective danger.[135] As a result, a message which claims that vaccines cause very little risk may be less influential than negative information about very rare side effects, since people are cognitively biased toward negative reports. Additionally, people seem to "trust 'no risk' messages about vaccines less than messages stating the existence of risk."[136] Interestingly enough, "information stating the presence of risk decreases risk perceptions, while information negating the existence of risk increases such perceptions."[137] It is not necessarily helpful to try to completely deny that medical practices, such as vaccination, are entirely without risk. Strangely enough, that can actually increase perceptions of danger.

The Narrative bias reflects our propensity to mentally favour stories above facts. This includes preferencing people's testimonies and personal accounts of what they have experienced, rather than facts and statistics. Even if people know about the statistical scientific evidence around vaccine safety, hearing numerous narratives about apparent adverse vaccine outcomes can still lead to miscalculations about the risks associated with vaccine side effects.[138] This tendency is also tied to the negativity bias, because narratives with negatives plotlines about higher vaccination risks can have much stronger influences than might statistical information. There are numerous other cognitive biases, but these five represent some of the most instrumental cognitive tendencies to keep in mind when considering vaccine hesitancy. It is also important to remember that such biases influence everyone's thinking, so it is necessary to be aware of your own biased cognition as much as anyone else's. Finally, consider this: If everyone is influenced by the subtle psychology of biases, might there be ways for pro-vaccine advocacy to work *with* such cognitive biases rather than attempting to fight against them?

Starting strong: Guidelines to build upon

Asking whether pro-vaccine advocacy could be improved by working with biases, rather than against them, is not only practical but it also involves questioning whether vaccine promotion can possibly be enhanced. This is a vital consideration because, as has been noted in this chapter, responding to vaccine hesitancy, and trying to modify vaccination behaviours, appear to be particularly challenging. To address this challenge, it is important to start advocacy strong by taking into account the five general guidelines discussed above, which include such fundamentals as remaining audience-focussed, employing Motivational Interviewing, and being willing to acknowledge people's fears. Remember too that listening is a vital skill, which can be developed through the HURIER model. Potential behaviour-modification techniques, such as choice architecture, and the importance of healthcare provider interactions should also be taken into account. Vaccine advocacy may further be improved by addressing cultural cognition, affirming autonomy of choice, and being mindful of biases. The next chapter will add an additional framework of recommendations for improving vaccine advocacy by building upon this preliminary advice. It will do so by first explaining why it is best to focus on vaccine hesitant "fence-sitters" rather than ardent vaccine deniers, while identifying the need to tailor advocacy for specific audiences. The chapter will also introduce better debunking techniques and outline simple ways of making vaccine facts stickier.

Notes

1　Amanda F. Dempsey et al., "Characteristics of Users of a Tailored, Interactive Website for Parents and Its Impact on Adolescent Vaccination Attitudes and Uptake," *BMC Research Notes* 8, no. 1 (2015); Mirjam Pot et al., "Effectiveness of a Web-Based Tailored Intervention with Virtual Assistants Promoting the Acceptability of HPV Vaccination among Mothers of Invited Girls: Randomized Controlled Trial," *Journal of Medical Internet Research* 19, no. 9 (2017); Glen J. Nowak et al., "Using Immersive Virtual Reality to Improve the Beliefs and Intentions of Influenza Vaccine Avoidant 18-to-49-Year-Olds: Considerations, Effects, and Lessons Learned," *Vaccine* 38, no. 5 (2020); Glen J. Nowak, Angela K. Shen, and Jason L. Schwartz, "Using Campaigns to Improve Perceptions of the Value of Adult Vaccination in the United States: Health Communication Considerations and Insights," *Vaccine* 35, no. 42 (2017).

2　Brendan Nyhan and Jason Reifler, "Does Correcting Myths About the Flu Vaccine Work? An Experimental Evaluation of the Effects of Corrective

Information," *Vaccine* 33, no. 3 (2015); Sara Pluviano et al., "Parents' Beliefs in Misinformation About Vaccines Are Strengthened by Pro-Vaccine Campaigns," *Cogn Process* 20, no. 3 (2019); Sara Pluviano, Caroline Watt, and Sergio Della Sala, "Misinformation Lingers in Memory: Failure of Three Pro-Vaccination Strategies," *PLoS One* 12, no. 7 (2017); Ali M. Shropshire, Renee Brent-Hotchkiss, and Urkovia K. Andrews, "Mass Media Campaign Impacts Influenza Vaccine Obtainment of University Students," *J Am Coll Health* 61, no. 8 (2013).

3   Noel T. Brewer et al., "Increasing Vaccination: Putting Psychological Science into Action," *Psychological Science in the Public Interest* 18, no. 3 (2017): 186–87; Brendan Nyhan et al., "Effective Messages in Vaccine Promotion: A Randomized Trial," *Pediatrics* 133, no. 4 (2014).

4   Allison Kempe et al., "Physician Response to Parental Requests to Spread out the Recommended Vaccine Schedule," *Pediatrics* 135 (2015).

5   Eve Dubé, Dominique Gagnon, and Noni E. MacDonald, "Strategies Intended to Address Vaccine Hesitancy: Review of Published Reviews," *Vaccine* 33, no. 34 (2015): 4200.

6   IGA, "Section 1220.403 Dentists Administering Flu Vaccines," Ilinois General Assembly, https://www.ilga.gov/commission/jcar/admincode/068/068012200D04030R.html; OBD, "Oregon Board of Dentistry – Vaccine Information," https://www.oregon.gov/dentistry/Documents/Oregon%20Boa rd%20of%20Dentistry%20Vaccine%20Information.pdf; BDA, "Scotland: Dentists Can Give Flu Vaccinations This Winter," https://bda.org/news-centre/la test-news-articles/Pages/Scotland-Dentists-can-give-flu-vaccinations-this-winter. aspx; NCIRS, "Vaccination from Community Pharmacy," https://www.ncirs. org.au/public/vaccination-community-pharmacy.

7   Bridget Haire et al., "Raising Rates of Childhood Vaccination: The Trade-Off between Coercion and Trust," *Journal of Bioethical Inquiry* 15, no. 2 (2018).

8   Rawan Nour, "A Systematic Review of Methods to Improve Attitudes Towards Childhood Vaccinations," *Cureus* 11, no. 7 (2019).

9   Paul L. Reiter, Melissa B. Gilkey, and Noel T. Brewer, "HPV Vaccination among Adolescent Males: Results from the National Immunization Survey-Teen," *Vaccine* 31, no. 26 (2013); Elisabetta Pandolfi et al., "The Effect of Physician's Recommendation on Seasonal Influenza Immunization in Children with Chronic Diseases," *BMC Public Health* 12, no. 1 (2012); Kerrie E. Wiley and Julie Leask, "Respiratory Vaccine Uptake During Pregnancy," *The Lancet* 1, no. 1 (2013); Philip J. Smith et al., "Association between Health Care Providers' Influence on Parents Who Have Concerns About Vaccine Safety and Vaccination Coverage," *Pediatrics* 118, no. 5 (2006); Kathryn M. Edwards and Jesse M. Hackell, "Countering Vaccine Hesitancy," *Pediatrics* 138, no. 3 (2016); Kristen L. Myers, "Predictors of Maternal Vaccination in the United States: An Integrative Review of the Literature," *Vaccine* 34, no. 34 (2016); Douglas J. Opel et al., "The Architecture of Provider-Parent Vaccine Discussions at Health Supervision Visits," *Pediatrics* 132, no. 6 (2013).

10   Haire et al., "Raising Rates of Childhood Vaccination: The Trade-Off between Coercion and Trust."

11   Allison Kempe et al., "Prevalence of Parental Concerns About Childhood Vaccines: The Experience of Primary Care Physicians," *American Journal of Preventive Medicine* 40, no. 5 (2011).

12   Amanda F. Dempsey and Gregory D. Zimet, "Interventions to Improve Adolescent Vaccination: What May Work and What Still Needs to Be Tested," *American Journal of Preventive Medicine* 49, no. 6 (2015).

13   John Cook, Daniel Bedford, and Scott Mandia, "Raising Climate Literacy through Addressing Misinformation: Case Studies in Agnotology-Based

Learning," *Journal of Geoscience Education* 62, no. 3 (2014); Radomír Masaryk and Mária Hatoková, "Qualitative Inquiry into Reasons Why Vaccination Messages Fail," *Journal of Health Psychology* 22, no. 14 (2017).

14   P. Sol Hart and Erik C. Nisbet, "Boomerang Effects in Science Communication: How Motivated Reasoning and Identity Cues Amplify Opinion Polarization About Climate Mitigation Policies," *Communication Research* 39, no. 6 (2012).

15   Douglas S. Diekema, "Improving Childhood Vaccination Rates," *The New England Journal of Medicine* 366, no. 5 (2012): 392.

16   Mike Klymkowsky, "What Can the Anti-Vaccination Movement Teach Us About Improving the Public's Understanding of Science?," *PhysOrg*, https://phys. org/news/2017-01-anti-vaccination-movement-science.html.

17   Catherine C. McClure, Jessica R. Cataldi, and Sean T. O'Leary, "Vaccine Hesitancy: Where We Are and Where We Are Going," *Clinical Therapeutics* 39, no. 8 (2017); Heidi J. Larson et al., "Addressing the Vaccine Confidence Gap," *Lancet* 378, no. 9790 (2011); Jacquelin R. Meszaros et al., "Cognitive Processes and the Decisions of Some Parents to Forego Pertussis Vaccination for Their Children," *Journal of Clinical Epidemiology* 49, no. 6 (1996).

18   Seth Mnookin, *The Panic Virus: Fear, Myth and the Vaccination Debate* (New York: Simon and Schuster, 2011), 10.

19   Nyhan and Reifler, "Does Correcting Myths About the Flu Vaccine Work? An Experimental Evaluation of the Effects of Corrective Information"; Dan Kahan et al., "Motivated Numeracy and Enlightened Self-Government," *Behavioural Public Policy* 1, no. 1 (2017): 78–79; Angus Thomson, Karis Robinson, and Gaëlle Vallée-Tourangeau, "The 5as: A Practical Taxonomy for the Determinants of Vaccine Uptake," *Vaccine* 34, no. 8 (2016): 1022.

20   Andrea L. Benin et al., "Qualitative Analysis of Mothers' Decision-Making About Vaccines for Infants: The Importance of Trust," *Pediatrics* 117, no. 5 (2006); Melissa L. Carrion, "An Ounce of Prevention: Identifying Cues to (in) Action for Maternal Vaccine Refusal," *Qualitative Health Research* 28, no. 14 (2018); Catherine Helps et al., "Understanding Non-Vaccinating Parents' Views to Inform and Improve Clinical Encounters: A Qualitative Study in an Australian Community," *BMJ* 9, no. 5 (2019).

21   Michael G. Anderson et al., "A Clinical Perspective of the U.S. Anti-Vaccination Epidemic: Considering Marginal Costs and Benefits, CDC Best Practices Guidelines, Free Riders, and Herd Immunity," *Vaccine* 38, no. 50 (2020); A. Kroger, L. Bahta, S. Long and P. Sanchez, "General Best Practice Guidelines for Immunization. Best Practices Guidance of the Advisory Committee on Immunization Practices (ACIP)," CDC, https://www.cdc.gov/vaccines/ hcp/acip-recs/general-recs/downloads/general-recs.pdf.

22   M. C. Beach, "Do Patients Treated with Dignity Report Higher Satisfaction, Adherence, and Receipt of Preventive Care?," *Annals of Family Medicine* 3, no. 4 (2005): 337.

23   Arnaud Gagneur et al., "A Postpartum Vaccination Promotion Intervention Using Motivational Interviewing Techniques Improves Short-Term Vaccine Coverage: Promovac Study," *BMC Public Health* 18, no. 1 (2018); Thomas Lemaitre et al., "Impact of a Vaccination Promotion Intervention Using Motivational Interview Techniques on Long-Term Vaccine Coverage: The Promovac Strategy," *Human Vaccines & Immunotherapeutic* 15, no. 3 (2019); Anne E. Stocker et al., "Motivational Interviewing and Vaccinations in Pediatric Practice," *International Journal of Child Health and Human Development* 14, no. 1 (2021); Lucas A. Berenbrok et al., "Impact of Pharmacist Motivational Interviewing on Hepatitis B Vaccination in Adults with Diabetes," *Journal of the American Pharmacists Association* 63, no. 1 (2022); Kim C. Coley et

al., "Increasing Adult Vaccinations at a Regional Supermarket Chain Pharmacy: A Multi-Site Demonstration Project," *Vaccine* 38, no. 24 (2020); Amber PharmD Brackett, Michell PharmD Butler, and Liza PharmD Chapman, "Using Motivational Interviewing in the Community Pharmacy to Increase Adult Immunization Readiness: A Pilot Evaluation," *Journal of the American Pharmacists Association* 55, no. 2 (2015); Zixin Wang et al., "Two Web-Based and Theory-Based Interventions with and without Brief Motivational Interviewing in the Promotion of Human Papillomavirus Vaccination among Chinese Men Who Have Sex with Men: Randomized Controlled Trial," *Journal of Medical Internet Research* 23, no. 2 (2021); Arnaud Gagneur et al., "Promoting Vaccination in Maternity Wards – Motivational Interview Technique Reduces Hesitancy and Enhances Intention to Vaccinate, Results from a Multicentre Non-Controlled Pre- and Post-Intervention RCT-nested Study, Quebec, March 2014 to February 2015," *Eurosurveillance* 24, no. 36 (2019); Arnaud Gagneur, Virginie Gosselin, and Ève Dubé, "Motivational Interviewing: A Promising Tool to Address Vaccine Hesitancy," *Vaccine* 36, no. 44 (2018); Amanda F. Dempsey et al., "Effect of a Health Care Professional Communication Training Intervention on Adolescent Human Papillomavirus Vaccination: A Cluster Randomized Clinical Trial," *JAMA Pediatrics* 172, no. 5 (2018).

24 Stephen Rollnick, William R. Miller, and Christopher Butler, *Motivational Interviewing in Health Care: Helping Patients Change Behavior* (New York: Guilford Press, 2008).

25 Ibid., 6.

26 Ibid., 6–7.

27 Ibid., 7.

28 William R. Miller and Stephen Rollnick, *Motivational Interviewing: Preparing People for Change*, 2nd ed. (New York: Guilford Press, 2002), 65.

29 Monica Zolezzi, Bridget Paravattil, and Taysier El-Gaili, "Using Motivational Interviewing Techniques to Inform Decision-Making for COVID-19 Vaccination," *International Journal of Clinical Pharmacy* 43, no. 6 (2021): 1729.

30 Adapted from Loren Bonner, "COVID-19 Provides Opportunity to Rethink Vaccine Hesitancy," *Pharmacy Today* 27, no. 5 (2021): 30.

31 Arnaud Gagneur, "Motivational Interviewing: A Powerful Tool to Address Vaccine Hesitancy," *Canada Communicable Disease Report* 46, no. 4 (2020): 95.

32 Zolezzi, Paravattil, and El-Gaili, "Using Motivational Interviewing Techniques to Inform Decision-Making for COVID-19 Vaccination," 1729.

33 Adapted from ibid.

34 Gagneur, "Motivational Interviewing: A Powerful Tool to Address Vaccine Hesitancy," 96.

35 Zolezzi, Paravattil, and El-Gaili, "Using Motivational Interviewing Techniques to Inform Decision-Making for COVID-19 Vaccination," 1729.

36 Gagneur, "Motivational Interviewing: A Powerful Tool to Address Vaccine Hesitancy," 96.

37 Judi Brownell, "The Skills of Listening-Centered Communication," in *Listening and Human Communication in the 21st Century*, ed. Andrew D. Wolvin (Oxford: Wiley-Blackwell, 2010).

38 Judi Brownell, *Listening: Attitudes, Principles, and Skills*, Sixth ed. (New York, NY: Routledge, 2016), 70.

39 Ibid., 15.

40 Ibid., 12.

41 Adapted from ibid.

42 Judi Brownell, "Exploring the Strategic Ground for Listening and Organizational Effectiveness," *Scandinavian Journal of Hospitality and Tourism* 8, no. 3 (2008): 218.

43   Brownell, "The Skills of Listening-Centered Communication," 144.
44   Ibid., 145.
45   Brownell, *Listening: Attitudes, Principles, and Skills*, 112–14.
46   Ibid., 115.
47   Brownell, "The Skills of Listening-Centered Communication," 145.
48   Brownell, *Listening: Attitudes, Principles, and Skills*, 148.
49   Ibid., 13.
50   Ibid., 172.
51   Brownell, "The Skills of Listening-Centered Communication," 146.
52   Brownell, "Exploring the Strategic Ground for Listening and Organizational Effectiveness," 219.
53   Ibid.
54   Brownell, *Listening: Attitudes, Principles, and Skills*, 223.
55   Brownell, "The Skills of Listening-Centered Communication," 146.
56   Brownell, *Listening: Attitudes, Principles, and Skills*, 261.
57   Ibid., 22.
58   Scott A. Myers, "Perceived Instructor Credibility and Verbal Aggressiveness in the College Classroom," *Communication Research Reports* 18, no. 4 (2001): 354.
59   A. Harnden and J. Shakespeare, "10-Minute Consultation: MMR Immunisation," *BMJ* 323, no. 7303 (2001); Rosemary J. Burnett et al., "Addressing Public Questioning and Concerns About Vaccination in South Africa: A Guide for Healthcare Workers," *Vaccine* 30, no. 3 (2012); Vidya Bhushan Gupta, "Communicating with Parents of Children with Autism About Vaccines and Complementary and Alternative Approaches," *Journal of Developmental & Behavioral Pediatrics* 31, no. 4 (2010); Cornelia Betsch and Katharina Sachse, "Dr. Jekyll or Mr. Hyde? (How) the Internet Influences Vaccination Decisions: Recent Evidence and Tentative Guidelines for Online Vaccine Communication," *Vaccine* 30, no. 25 (2012): 3724.
60   Joshua Greenberg, Eve Dubé, and Michelle Driedger, "Vaccine Hesitancy: In Search of the Risk Communication Comfort Zone," *PLoS Currents* 9 (2017); Cornelia Betsch, "Innovations in Communication: The Internet and the Psychology of Vaccination Decisions," *Eurosurveillance* 16, no. 17 (2011); Amanda Dempsey, "Communicating with Families About HPV," *Journal of Clinical Outcomes Management* 24, no. 3 (2017).
61   Myers, "Perceived Instructor Credibility and Verbal Aggressiveness in the College Classroom"; Kjerstin Thorson, Emily Vraga, and Brian Ekdale, "Credibility in Context: How Uncivil Online Commentary Affects News Credibility," *Mass Communication & Society* 13, no. 3 (2010).
62   Scott A. Myers, "Perceived Aggressive Instructor Communication and Student State Motivation, Learning, and Satisfaction," *Communication Reports* 15, no. 2 (2002); Yang Lin, James M. Durbin, and Andrew S. Rancer, "Perceived Instructor Argumentativeness, Verbal Aggressiveness, and Classroom Communication Climate in Relation to Student State Motivation and Math Anxiety," *Communication Education* 66, no. 3 (2017); Shupei Yuan, John C. Besley, and Wenjuan Ma, "Be Mean or Be Nice? Understanding the Effects of Aggressive and Polite Communication Styles in Child Vaccination Debate," *Health Communication* 34, no. 10 (2018).
63   Heidi J. Larson et al., "Measuring Trust in Vaccination: A Systematic Review," *Human Vaccines & Immunotherapeutics* 14, no. 7 (2018); Heidi J. Larson et al., "Understanding Vaccine Hesitancy around Vaccines and Vaccination from a Global Perspective: A Systematic Review of Published Literature, 2007–2012," *Vaccine* 32, no. 19 (2014).
64   Roi Piñeiro Pérez et al., "Vaccination Counselling: The Meeting Point Is Possible," *Anales de Pediatría* 86, no. 6 (2017): 317.

65 A. Reich Jennifer, *Calling the Shots* (New York: New York University Press, 2016), 240–41.

66 Claire Hooker, "How to Cut through When Talking to Anti-Vaxxers and Anti-Fluoriders," *The Conversation*, https://theconversation.com/how-to-cut-through-when-talking-to-anti-vaxxers-and-anti-fluoriders-72504.

67 Anna Kata, "A Postmodern Pandora's Box: Anti-Vaccination Misinformation on the Internet," *Vaccine* 28, no. 7 (2010): 36–41.

68 Leah Ceccarelli, "Manufactured Scientific Controversy: Science, Rhetoric, and Public Debate," *Rhetoric and Public Affairs* 14, no. 2 (2011).

69 B. H. Levi, "Addressing Parents' Concerns About Childhood Immunizations: A Tutorial for Primary Care Providers," *Pediatrics* 120, no. 1 (2007).

70 Richard M. Carpiano and Nicholas S. Fitz, "Public Attitudes toward Child Undervaccination: A Randomized Experiment on Evaluations, Stigmatizing Orientations, and Support for Policies," *Social Science & Medicine* 185 (2017); Masaryk and Hatoková, "Qualitative Inquiry into Reasons Why Vaccination Messages Fail."; Dan Kahan, "A Risky Science Communication Environment for Vaccines," *Science* 342, no. 6154 (2013); Julie Leask, "Should We Do Battle with Antivaccination Activists?," *Public Health Research & Practice* 25, no. 2 (2015).

71 K. M. Edwards and J. M. Hackell, "Countering Vaccine Hesitancy," *Pediatrics* 138, no. 3 (2016): 7.

72 Frank H. Beard et al., "Trends and Patterns in Vaccination Objection, Australia, 2002–2013," *Medical Journal of Australia* 204, no. 7 (2016).

73 Meng Li and Gretchen B. Chapman, "Nudge to Health: Harnessing Decision Research to Promote Health Behavior: Nudge to Health," *Social and Personality Psychology Compass* 7, no. 3 (2013): 192; Rachel Caskey et al., "A Behavioral Economic Approach to Improving Human Papillomavirus Vaccination," *Journal of Adolescent Health* 61, no. 6 (2017); Florian H. Schneider et al., "Financial Incentives for Vaccination Do Not Have Negative Unintended Consequences," *Nature* (2023).

74 V. Paul-Ebhohimhen and A. Avenell, "Systematic Review of the Use of Financial Incentives in Treatments for Obesity and Overweight," *Obesity Reviews* 9, no. 4 (2008); Carwyn Langdown and Stephen Peckham, "The Use of Financial Incentives to Help Improve Health Outcomes: Is the Quality and Outcomes Framework Fit for Purpose? A Systematic Review," *Journal of Public Health* 36, no. 2 (2014).

75 Craig Smith, Claire Duffy, and Michelle Kirszner, *Research to Identify Immunisation Information Needs: Qualitative Research Report* (Crows Nest: Department of Health, 2016), 26.

76 Gareth J. Hollands et al., "Altering Micro-Environments to Change Population Health Behaviour: Towards an Evidence Base for Choice Architecture Interventions," *BMC Public Health* 13, no. 1 (2013): 3.

77 Ibid., 2.

78 Richard H. Thaler and Cass R. Sunstein, *Nudge: Improving Decisions About Health, Wealth, and Happiness* (New Haven & London: Yale University Press, 2008), 6.

79 Ibid., 3–4.

80 Douglas J. Opel and Saad B. Omer, "Measles, Mandates, and Making Vaccination the Default Option," *JAMA Pediatrics* 169, no. 4 (2015).

81 Frej Klem Thomsen, "Childhood Immunization, Vaccine Hesitancy, and Provaccination Policy in High-Income Countries," *Psychology, Public Policy, and Law* 23, no. 3 (2017); McClure, Cataldi, and O'Leary, "Vaccine Hesitancy: Where We Are and Where We Are Going," 1557.

82 Greenberg, Dubé, and Driedger, "Vaccine Hesitancy: In Search of the Risk Communication Comfort Zone."

83   Michael Favin et al., "Why Children Are Not Vaccinated: A Review of the Grey Literature," *International Health* 4, no. 4 (2012); Linda Y. Fu et al., "Associations of Trust and Healthcare Provider Advice with HPV Vaccine Acceptance among African American Parents," *Vaccine* 35, no. 5 (2016); Pandolfi et al., "The Effect of Physician's Recommendation on Seasonal Influenza Immunization in Children with Chronic Diseases"; Smith et al., "Association between Health Care Providers' Influence on Parents Who Have Concerns About Vaccine Safety and Vaccination Coverage"; Reiter, Gilkey, and Brewer, "HPV Vaccination among Adolescent Males"; Wiley and Leask, "Respiratory Vaccine Uptake During Pregnancy."

84   D. A. Gust et al., "Parents with Doubts About Vaccines: Which Vaccines and Reasons Why," *Pediatrics* 122, no. 4 (2008).

85   Marissa Wheeler and Alison M. Buttenheim, "Parental Vaccine Concerns, Information Source, and Choice of Alternative Immunization Schedules," *Human Vaccines & Immunotherapeutics* 9, no. 8 (2013).

86   Opel et al., "The Architecture of Provider-Parent Vaccine Discussions at Health Supervision Visits."

87   Noel T. Brewer et al., "Announcements Versus Conversations to Improve HPV Vaccination Coverage: A Randomized Trial," *Pediatrics* 139, no. 1 (2017).

88   Ibid.

89   John C. Hershey et al., "The Roles of Altruism, Free Riding, and Bandwagoning in Vaccination Decisions," *Organizational Behavior and Human Decision Processes* 59, no. 2 (1994).

90   Alison M. Buttenheim and David A. Asch, "Making Vaccine Refusal Less of a Free Ride," *Human Vaccines & Immunotherapeutics* 9, no. 12 (2013): 2675.

91   McClure, Cataldi, and O'Leary, "Vaccine Hesitancy: Where We Are and Where We Are Going"; Meszaros et al., "Cognitive Processes and the Decisions of Some Parents to Forego Pertussis Vaccination for Their Children"; Ross D. Silverman and Lindsay F. Wiley, "Shaming Vaccine Refusal," *The Journal of Law, Medicine & Ethics* 45, no. 4 (2017).

92   Patti Williams, Gavan J. Fitzsimmons, and Lauren G. Block, "When Consumers Do Not Recognize 'Benign' Intention Questions as Persuasion Attempts," *Journal of Consumer Research* 31, no. 3 (2004): 540.

93   Ibid., 549–50.

94   Peter M. Gollwitzer and Paschal Sheeran, "Implementation Intentions and Goal Achievement: A Meta-Analysis of Effects and Processes," *Advances in Experimental Social Psychology* 38 (2006); Katherine L. Milkman et al., "Using Implementation Intentions Prompts to Enhance Influenza Vaccination Rates," *Proceedings of the National Academy of Sciences USA* 108, no. 26 (2011).

95   Jacob Heller, "Trust in Institutions, Science and Self – the Case of Vaccines," *Narrative Inquiry in Bioethics* 6, no. 3 (2016).

96   Anna Winterbottom et al., "Does Narrative Information Bias Individual's Decision Making? A Systematic Review," *Social Science & Medicine* 67, no. 12 (2008); Rachel M. Cunningham and Julie A. Boom, "Telling Stories of Vaccine-Preventable Diseases: Why It Works," *South Dakota Medicine* (2013).

97   Chingching Chang, "Increasing Mental Health Literacy via Narrative Advertising," *Journal of Health Communication* 13, no. 1 (2008); Adebanke L. Adebayo et al., "The Effectiveness of Narrative Versus Didactic Information Formats on Pregnant Women's Knowledge, Risk Perception, Self-Efficacy, and Information Seeking Related to Climate Change Health Risks," *International Journal of Environmental Research and Public Health* 17, no. 19 (2020); John B. F. de Wit, Enny Das, and Raymond Vet, "What Works Best: Objective Statistics or a Personal Testimonial? An Assessment of the Persuasive Effects of

Different Types of Message Evidence on Risk Perception," *Health Psychology* 27, no. 1 (2008).

98   Kenneth Holler and Anthony Scalzo, "'I've Heard Some Things That Scare Me'. Responding with Empathy to Parents' Fears of Vaccinations," *Missouri Medicine* 109, no. 1 (2012); Luz Martínez Martínez et al., "Formulas for Prevention, Narrative Versus Non-Narrative Formats. A Comparative Analysis of Their Effects on Young People's Knowledge, Attitude and Behaviour in Relation to HPV," *Revista Latina de Comunicación Social*, no. 73 (2018); Ubaldo Cuesta, Luz Martínez, and Victoria Cuesta, "Effectiveness of Narrative Persuasion on Facebook: Change of Attitude and Intention Towards HPV," *European Journal of Social Science Education and Research* 4, no. 6 (2017).

99   Dan Kahan, Hank Jenkins-Smith, and Donald Braman, "Cultural Cognition of Scientific Consensus," *Journal of Risk Research* 14, no. 2 (2011).

100 Richard Zimmerman et al., "Vaccine Criticism on the World Wide Web," *Journal of Medical Internet Research* 7, no. 2 (2005); McClure, Cataldi, and O'Leary, "Vaccine Hesitancy: Where We Are and Where We Are Going."

101 Deborah K. Johnson et al., "Combating Vaccine Hesitancy with Vaccine-Preventable Disease Familiarization: An Interview and Curriculum Intervention for College Students," *Vaccines* 7, no. 2 (2019).

102 Ibid., 10.

103 Ibid., 12.

104 Jacqueline Pich, "Patient Reminder and Recall Interventions to Improve Immunization Rates: A Cochrane Review Summary," *International Journal of Nursing Studies* 91 (2019); Sorelle N. Jones Cooper and Benita Walton-Moss, "Using Reminder/Recall Systems to Improve Influenza Immunization Rates in Children with Asthma," *Journal of Pediatric Health Care* 27, no. 5 (2013); Peter G. Szilagyi et al., "Effect of Patient Reminder/Recall Interventions on Immunization Rates: A Review," *JAMA* 284, no. 14 (2000); Gretchen J. Domek et al., "SMS Text Message Reminders to Improve Infant Vaccination Coverage in Guatemala: A Pilot Randomized Controlled Trial," *Vaccine* 34, no. 21 (2016); Elyse Olshen Kharbanda et al., "Text Message Reminders to Promote Human Papillomavirus Vaccination," *Vaccine* 29, no. 14 (2011).

105 Dan Kahan, "Fixing the Communications Failure," *Nature* 463, no. 7279 (2010).

106 "Misconceptions, Misinformation, and the Logic of Identity-Protective Cognition," *Cultural Cognition Project Working Paper Series*, no. 164 (2017).

107 "Ideology, Motivated Reasoning, and Cognitive Reflection," *Judgment and Decision Making* 8, no. 4 (2013); Thomas Wood and Ethan Porter, "The Elusive Backfire Effect: Mass Attitudes' Steadfast Factual Adherence," *Political Behavior* 41, no. 1 (2018).

108 Dan Kahan, "Cultural Cognition as a Conception of the Cultural Theory of Risk," in *Handbook of Risk Theory: Epistemology, Decision Theory, Ethics, and Social Implications of Risk*, ed. Sabine Roeser, et al. (Dordrecht: Springer, 2012), 753.

109 Ibid., 752.

110 Ibid., 752–53.

111 Adapted from ibid., 732.

112 Dan Kahan, "Making Climate-Science Communication Evidence-Based: All the Way Down," in *Culture, Politics and Climate Change: How Information Shapes Our Common Future*, ed. Deserai A. Crow and Maxwell T. Boykoff (Abingdon: Routledge, 2014).

113 Kahan, "Cultural Cognition," 753.

114 Ibid.

115 Ibid.

116 Kahan, "Fixing the Communications Failure," 297.
117 Ibid.
118 Kahan, "Cultural Cognition," 752.
119 Ibid.
120 Dan Kahan et al., "Who Fears the HPV Vaccine, Who Doesn't, and Why?: An Experimental Study of the Mechanisms of Cultural Cognition," *Law and Human Behavior* 34, no. 6 (2010): 513.
121 Dan Kahan et al., "Culture and Identity-Protective Cognition: Explaining the White-Male Effect in Risk Perception," *Journal of Empirical Legal Studies* 4, no. 3 (2007): 36.
122 Helps et al., "Understanding Non-Vaccinating Parents' Views to Inform and Improve Clinical Encounters: A Qualitative Study in an Australian Community," 5–6; Matthew J. Hornsey, Emily A. Harris, and Kelly S. Fielding, "The Psychological Roots of Anti-Vaccination Attitudes: A 24-Nation Investigation," *Health Psychology* 37, no. 4 (2018).
123 Haire et al., "Raising Rates of Childhood Vaccination: The Trade-Off between Coercion and Trust."
124 Harnden and Shakespeare, "10-Minute Consultation: MMR Immunisation."
125 J. Leask et al., "Communicating with Parents About Vaccination: A Framework for Health Professionals," *BMC Pediatrics* 12, no. 1 (2012).
126 Brownell, "The Skills of Listening-Centered Communication," 144.
127 OED, "*Bias, V.2a*" (Oxford University Press).
128 Brownell, "Exploring the Strategic Ground for Listening and Organizational Effectiveness," 219.
129 Kerri A. Goodwin and C. James Goodwin, *Research in Psychology: Methods and Design*, 8th ed. (Hoboken, NJ: Wiley, 2017), 6; Raymond S. Nickerson, "Confirmation Bias: A Ubiquitous Phenomenon in Many Guises," *Review of General Psychology* 2, no. 2 (1998).
130 Gary D. Sherman et al., "When Taking Action Means Accepting Responsibility: Omission Bias Predicts Parents' Reluctance to Vaccinate Due to Greater Anticipated Culpability for Negative Side Effects," *Journal of Consumer Affairs* 55, no. 4 (2021).
131 David A. Asch et al., "Omission Bias and Pertussis Vaccination," *Medical Decision Making* 14, no. 2 (1994); Meszaros et al., "Cognitive Processes and the Decisions of Some Parents to Forego Pertussis Vaccination for Their Children"; Katrina F. Brown et al., "Omission Bias and Vaccine Rejection by Parents of Healthy Children: Implications for the Influenza a/H1N1 Vaccination Programme," *Vaccine* 28, no. 25 (2010); Caitlin E. Hansen, Anna North, and Linda M. Niccolai, "Cognitive Bias in Clinicians' Communication About Human Papillomavirus Vaccination," *Health Communication* 35, no. 4 (2020); Helena Tomljenovic, Andreja Bubic, and Nikola Erceg, "Contribution of Rationality to Vaccine Attitudes: Testing Two Hypotheses," *Journal of Behavioral Decision Making* 35, no. 2 (2022); Julie A. PhD M. P. H. Bettinger, Devon PhD Greyson, and Deborah M. D. Money, "Attitudes and Beliefs of Pregnant Women and New Mothers Regarding Influenza Vaccination in British Columbia," *Journal of Obstetrics and Gynaecology Canada* 38, no. 11 (2016); Christine L. Lackner and Charles H. Wang, "Demographic, Psychological, and Experiential Correlates of SARS-CoV-2 Vaccination Intentions in a Sample of Canadian Families," *Vaccine X* 8 (2021).
132 Marco daCosta DiBonaventura and Gretchen B. Chapman, "Do Decision Biases Predict Bad Decisions? Omission Bias, Naturalness Bias, and Influenza Vaccination," *Medical Decision Making* 28, no. 4 (2008): 533.
133 Asami Yagi, Yutaka Ueda, and Tadashi Kimura, "A Behavioral Economics Approach to the Failed HPV Vaccination Program in Japan," *Vaccine* 35, no. 50 (2017).

134 Sherry L. Seethaler, "Shades of Grey in Vaccination Decision Making: Tradeoffs, Heuristics, and Implications," *Science Communication* 38, no. 2 (2016): 264.

135 Michael Siegrist and George Cvetkovich, "Better Negative Than Positive? Evidence of a Bias for Negative Information About Possible Health Dangers," *Risk Analysis* 21, no. 1 (2001).

136 Cornelia Betsch and Katharina Sachse, "Debunking Vaccination Myths: Strong Risk Negations Can Increase Perceived Vaccination Risks," *Health Psychology* 32, no. 2 (2013): 147.

137 Ibid., 146.

138 Betsch Cornelia et al., "The Narrative Bias Revisited: What Drives the Biasing Influence of Narrative Information on Risk Perceptions?," *Judgment and Decision Making* 10, no. 3 (2015).

6   Better advocacy

Debunking and sticky facts

In 2018, the Independent Investigations Group at the Center for Inquiry invited several flat-earthers to the Salton Sea in California. The investigations team met up with the spherical earth deniers to conduct two straightforward round-earth experiments. These tests would substantiate the planet's curvature while a National Geographic Explorer film crew was on hand to record the proceedings, and the flat-earthers' reactions.[1] As one of the world's largest inland seas and California's largest lake, the Salton Sea covers 970 square kilometres, making it a convenient place to conduct spherical-earth tests. The site was selected because flat-earthers insist that such large bodies of water are perfectly level, as they rest on a noncurved earth. Unsurprisingly, both experiments went as predicted if the earth is in fact a sphere.

The first of these tests attempted to view large helium-filled balloons through optical instruments from one side of the lake as they were released on the other shore. Due to the considerable size of the Salton Sea, the opposite shoreline was located approximately 14.5 kilometres across the water. It was predicted that the curvature of the earth would result in the balloons only being visible when they were floating several metres in the air. This is because the planet's arch would be sufficient enough to hide them from view until they had risen above a certain altitude. If the earth were flat, however, the observers would expect to see the balloons immediately through a telescope, without them needing to be raised far into the sky. The second test involved putting a boat carrying a large rectangular target out into Salton Sea. The target featured several 30cm thick horizontal stripes. In the case of a spherical earth, the stripes would recede below the lake horizon as the boat moved farther from shore. However, if the earth were flat, the experimenters would not observe the stripes disappearing as the boat travelled into the distance over a completely flat, uncurving body of water. In the end, the helium-filled balloons were only visible after they had risen approximately 13.7 meters into the air. As for the second experiment, one of the stripes on the boat target was almost completely below the horizon once the boat had travelled nearly 5 kilometres the from shore, and it could be observed receding due to the earth's curve. Both results empirically demonstrated that the planet was round.

DOI: 10.4324/9781003312550-6

One of the people on hand that day was Mark Sargent, a prominent flat-earth advocate, who was joined by several other ardent round-earth deniers. After the experiments were conducted, Sargent and the other flat-earthers rejected the results outright, claiming that other factors such as optical effects had truly caused the outcomes. The curvature of the planet was certainly *not* responsible for the Salton Sea observations. They also argued that the flat-earth reality was being covered up through a conspiracy. Ultimately, the flat-earth supporters concluded that the tests confirmed that the earth was in fact flat and not round. This anecdote is a lesson about how difficult it can be to change the minds of devoted science deniers. Regrettably, direct empirical evidence will usually not pierce the cultural cognition and conspiracy worldviews associated with such beliefs. Keeping this potentially disheartening fact in mind, the present chapter adds the final scaffolding of practical advice for improving vaccine advocacy. Building upon the five general guidelines introduced previously, it first considers the importance of directing attention to vaccine hesitant "fence-sitters" rather than ardent antivaccinationists. It discusses the need to tailor vaccine messages for specific audiences before exploring tips about how to more effectively debunk misinformation. This includes covering the idea of pre-bunking, or *Inoculation Theory*, prior to delving into how to make vaccination facts stickier.

Target fence-sitters and tailor messages

The Independent Investigations Group's round earth tests are characteristic of many interchanges that occur between experts and vaccine deniers. They also reveal why it has been recommended that pro-vaccine advocates should avoid trying to convert ardent vaccine rejectors. Unfortunately, fervent antivaccinationists are the least open to impartial argumentation and scientific evidence. Therefore, as with the flat earthers and the Salton Sea tests, expending energy to persuade ardent antivaccinationists is unlikely to be successful, either in person or online. Even though it can be tempting to engage antivaccine campaigners, trying to sway vocal deniers will most likely fail, as committed denial is resistant to evidence. Energy is better spent elsewhere. Recall also that ardent vaccine deniers represent comparatively small fractions of most nations' total populations, though they can be disproportionately media vocal and culturally influential.

Instead, attention should be given to so-called "fence-sitters," who are vaccine hesitant but undecided individuals, representing much larger segments of the public.[2] Fence-sitters can express a range of vaccine criticisms in the form of immunisation doubts and opinions. Nonetheless, they have not taken an altogether zealous side on the matter, even if they may have delayed or not fully conformed to official vaccination recommendations. Focusing on this larger, more ambivalent section of the population is strategic in terms of audience size and outcomes related to the time and effort needed to reach them. As one group of researchers put it, a vaccine spokesperson "should see it as his or her role to inform undecided individuals, equip vaccine advocates with evidence-based arguments and even convince sceptics."[3] However, vaccine advocates should "not be distracted by any ambition to convince the vaccine denier." There are further benefits to not addressing staunch antivaccinationists directly with arguments, in an effort to publicly discredit counter-immunisation groups. This is because, as one researcher concluded, focussing on counter-vaccine promoters could actually "give oxygen to antivaccination activists," and it may provide a form of legitimacy to their movement.[4] Targeting strident antivaccinationists can draw unnecessary attention to counter-immunisation leaders, and provoke "highly polarized discussions." This activity may also perpetuate "a false sense that vaccination is a highly contested topic," even though it is not a scientifically disputed issue.[5]

Researchers have further advised that science advocates tailor pro-vaccine communications for specific audiences. Some of the most persuasive public health messages are those that take into account the explicit informational needs, cultural contexts, and unique vaccine uncertainties maintained by particular groups of people whom they are attempting to reach.[6] For this reason, vaccination supporters are encouraged to gain insights into an audience's distinct attitudes and opinions, life experiences, interests, social values and personality traits, which may influence vaccination decisions. More effective vaccination messages can then be built around connecting with these qualities.[7] Such advice also relates to being aware of cultural cognition (Chapter 2), because a recommended goal of tailoring involves ensuring that pro-vaccination messages are compatible with people's cultural worldviews and social values.[8]

Tailoring communications "works by increasing the personal relevance of health messages."[9] In line with the Elaboration Likelihood model of persuasion (Chapter 2), when "individuals perceive information to be personally relevant, this may enhance their motivation to elaborate on the message."[10] Accordingly, tailoring communications can enhance a message's perceived personal meaning, which may also improve its persuasiveness. In short, this approach simply involves applying the tried-and-true adage of *knowing your audience*. Crucially, that audience should be the fence-sitters and not impassioned antivaccinationists.

Debunking I: Facts, repetition, and the truth sandwich

Vaccine advocacy can be further sharpened with improved debunking techniques used to tackle misinformation. The question is, what does effective debunking look like and what kinds of pro-vaccine methods work? In 2014, a group of researchers attempted to help answer such questions by testing the effectiveness of four types of vaccination messages, designed to improve people's intention to vaccinate their children with the

MMR vaccine.[11] The first strategy consisted of trying to correct vaccine misinformation. This involved presenting scientific evidence that debunked the widely discredited link between the MMR vaccine and autism (Chapter 4). The second method presented the facts about the risks associated with measles, mumps, and rubella. With this technique, symptoms and possible adverse events associated with the diseases were described. The third communication technique used a firsthand narrative. This involved recounting a mother's story about her child's hospitalisation due to measles. Finally, the fourth strategy employed visual images to express the risk of vaccine preventable diseases. The study's participants were shown pictures of children who suffered from either the measles, mumps, or rubella viruses.

Remarkably, the study found that *none* of the methods increased the intention to vaccinate for individuals who were the most opposed to vaccination. In fact, for some parents, the pro-vaccine communications increased their vaccine misperceptions, which resulted in lower intentions to vaccinate. Using a firsthand narrative about measles infection seemed to be counterproductive, and strangely "increased beliefs in the likelihood of serious side effects from MMR."[12] Showing people who already had unfavourable attitudes toward vaccines images of children with vaccine preventable diseases also appeared to intensify the belief that vaccines cause autism. When it came to communications that directly debunked links between the MMR vaccine and autism, the researchers explained:

> Among respondents with the least favorable attitudes toward vaccines, the predicted probability that respondents would be very likely to give MMR [to their children] decreased from 70% among control subjects to 45% for those given information debunking the supposed autism link.[13]

Attempts to debunk vaccine myths backfired and mysteriously strengthened erroneous beliefs for people who were already opposed to vaccination. When misinformation is dismantled for people, they can still go back to depending upon the debunked misinformation. This phenomenon has been named the *misinformation-persistence effect*, or the *continued influence effect* of misinformation.[14] It seems to be the result of people's "inability to update their memories in light of corrective information."[15] It also further reveals hitches in trying to convince those with the most negative opinions about vaccines.

What then can be done to improve attempts to debunk misinformation? The psychologists John Cook and Stephen Lewandowsky have attempted to help answer that question in detail.[16] One of the first debunking concerns that Cook and Lewandowsky considered is the *Familiarity Backfire Effect*, which is related to the results of the 2014 study discussed above. When attempts are made to try to debunk misinformation, the debunked myth must be mentioned so that an audience knows what false claims are being dealt with in the first place.[17] The problem is that when the mis-information is mentioned during debunking, people seem to become more familiar with the falsehood that they had already heard about. Some studies have found that over time audiences are more likely to recall, and to later believe in, restated misinformation instead of the facts, because they were more acquainted with the myth.[18] This may occur when pro-vaccine advocates endeavour to debunk the widespread myth that MMR vaccines cause autism. When the autism-vaccine myth is mentioned in order to discredit it, indivi-duals may lamentably end up remembering the misinformation instead of the genuine facts. Repeating myths, even when debunking them, could possibly improve people's memory recall of the more familiar misinformation.

In trying to understand these perplexing findings, more recent research has found that backfire effects are not necessarily as common as was once thought.[19] As a result, experts suggest that pro-vaccine advocates should not be overly worried about mentioning misinformation when trying to debunk myths.[20] Even so, needlessly repeating misinformation should still be avoi-ded, because it appears that "repetition makes information appear true."[21] This seems to be the case because of the way that our memories work, as well as the power of repetition in convincing listeners that something is accurate.[22] During World War 2, Floyd Allport and Milton Lepkin con-ducted a study to investigate why false wartime rumours persisted in the USA.[23] They found that the single best predictor of belief in a rumour was whether hearers had heard the rumour before on several occasions. More recent studies have contended that "simply repeating a statement causes it to be perceived as more valid or true."[24]

Importantly, it does not matter whether a repeated statement "is factually true, factually false, or an opinion; repetition enhances perceived validity for each."[25] This connection between repetition and message believability is known as the *Truth Effect*.[26] Its influence results from an increase in an audi-ence's familiarity with repeated claims. Statements that are more familiar seem more believable because audiences have heard them before, and so they are more accessible in people's memories, even when they are myths. In the end, the most important consideration is to begin debunking by emphasising the facts first, such as the reality that there is no scientific link between vaccines and autism, *before* a myth is mentioned.[27] Also, even though excessive caution about backfire effects is not warranted, it is beneficial to repeat facts multiple times and to conclude pro-vaccine advocacy with facts as well. Put simply, "The best approach is to focus on the facts you wish to communicate," and restating them rather than repeating myths unnecessarily.[28] Altogether, it is recommended that science advocates use the *truth sandwich* approach to debunking, which involves the following steps:[29]

1   *Fact*. State the truth right from the start.
2   *Myth*. Warn audiences about misinformation and mention the myth only once.

3   *Fallacy*. Explain what is wrong about the myth and reveal the mis-
    information's persuasion tactics.
4   *Fact*. Restate the genuine facts again.

This method captures the principal idea that pro-vaccine messages ought to
commence with facts rather than the myth being debunked, and they
should reinforce the facts at the very end. The truth sandwich approach is
also of use in *pre-bunking* efforts.

Debunking II: Pre-bunking and simplicity

When it comes to debunking, there is another valuable matter to consider,
which is described as pre-bunking or *Inoculation Theory*. Recall that vaccines
teach the immune system to fight infections from a pathogen by exposing it
to an antigen (Chapter 1). This trains the body and prepares it for exposure
to future disease threats. Intriguingly, researchers have discovered that it is
also possible to mentally inoculate people from the negative effects of antivaccination conspiracy theories. The idea is that presenting people with
common types of antivaccine persuasion tactics, as well as providing examples of misinformation arguments and their counterarguments, is cognitively
equivalent to giving individuals a weakened version of a pathogen via a
vaccine.[30] For example, Daniel Jolley and Karen Douglas found that if
individuals are presented with arguments against antivaccination conspiracy
theories prior to hearing about counter-vaccine conspiracies, it provides
people with a "means of defense, making them more resistant to persuasion
by conspiracy theories."[31] As they concluded, it appears that "combating
the potentially negative consequences of anti-vaccine conspiracy theories
may be achieved if people are exposed to accurate scientific information
before the conspiracy theories."[32]

The dilemma is that once people accept antivaccine conspiracies they are
extremely difficult to dislodge. Consequently, pre-bunking is far more
effective than attempting to debunk misinformation after individuals have
already accepted it. Notably, in many ways this book has been designed
around the benefits of pre-bunking. At its heart, the intent has been to
reveal common vaccine myths and their counterarguments, while uncovering the persuasion strategies exhibited throughout antivaccine messages.
The goal has not been to simply deliver more data, but to provide a suite
of insights, along with the tools required to inoculate people from future
exposure to misinformation. The hope is that by engaging with this book,
readers will be cognitively inoculated to numerous arguments, as well as
the tactics employed throughout antivaccine media and other types of
misinformation.

In the same vein as pre-bunking, it can be advantageous to forewarn
people about falsehoods before they are exposed to them, which is reflected
in Step 2 of the truth sandwich approach described above. Such warnings

"may induce a temporary state of skepticism and prompt the recipient to become more vigilant, and they may therefore be more likely to suppress misinformation."[33] It appears that the impact of repeating misinformation is lessened when people are warned *before* false information is mentioned.[34] Hence, if a myth is referred to in its debunking, it is advantageous to caution audiences beforehand that what they are about to hear is a scientifically invalidated claim.[35] It may also be helpful to forewarn listeners that "people tend to rely on misinformation even when it has been shown to be unreliable."[36]

Another invaluable piece of debunking advice is to make pro-vaccine messaging simple, easy to read, and understandable to non-specialists. This is because, "Information that is easy to process is more likely to be accepted as true."[37] Such guidance does not imply that advocates should stop using technical jargon, including complex health-related terms. Some specialised language signals to audiences that a communicator is an expert.[38] However, the goal should be to make pro-vaccine messages easier to grasp, read, and listen to, while still incorporating technical terminology when it is appropriate. Remember that part of the effectiveness of antivaccination media is that it is often written simply, with easy-to-understand arguments and stories.[39] That can make antivaccine messages less difficult to comprehend than more complicated pro-vaccine facts.

Comprehension may also be encouraged through the careful use of repetition. Repeating a few clearly stated phrases can make a message more memorable and easier to recall. In fact, it seems as though a simple and easy to understand myth is more psychologically appealing than are complicated, wordy debunking efforts.[40] The best communication recipe involves using short sentences and sticking to the facts.[41] Employing understandable and visually appealing graphics to make points is also effective. Finally, when ending a debunking message, finish with a clear-cut, uncomplicated message that is easy to remember. This may include such a statement as, "Scientific studies have found that MMR vaccines are safe." Debunkers are further reminded to be mindful of cognitive biases, such as the Confirmation bias (Chapter 5). In relation to this, keep in mind that people's worldviews can affect debunking.[42] From the perspective of the Cultural Cognition Thesis, this is why pro-vaccine advocates need to address cultural cognition, perhaps by applying cultural-identity affirmation as well as pluralistic advocacy.[43]

Finally, the most successful way to debunk misinformation is to ensure that a plausible, easily understood alternative for the myth being disproved is supplied.[44] This is because: "When you debunk a myth, you create a gap in the person's mind. To be effective, your debunking must fill that gap."[45] It is not simply enough to oppose misinformation, and pinpoint that it is false. The debunked misinformation must also be replaced with a credible narrative that serves as a substitute for the displaced myth. The need to replace misinformation with alternative facts has been described in the following way:

People build mental models of how the world works, where all the different parts of the model fit together like cogs. Imagine one of those cogs is a myth. When you explain that the myth is false, you pluck out that cog, leaving a gap in their mental model.

But people feel uncomfortable with an incomplete model. They want to feel as if they know what's going on. So if you create a gap, you need to fill the gap with an alternative fact.

For example, it's not enough to just provide evidence that a suspect in a murder trial is innocent. To prove them innocent – at least in people's minds – you need to provide an alternative suspect.[46]

If you do not fill the mental gap that debunking leaves behind with a credible and interesting fact, the myth may again be relied upon to restore the missing cog. This tendency is linked to the misinformation-persistence effect described above.[47] Alternatively, the gap left by a disproven myth can be filled by providing a possible explanation as to why someone would be spreading such misinformation, while exposing the persuasive techniques that are behind the debunked myth itself. This includes pointing out the types of persuasive cues that are being used in antivaccine messages, such as Source Cues, the Arousal of Fear, or the Scarcity Principle (chapters 3 and 4).

When all this advice is taken together, more effective debunking should endeavour to use the truth sandwich approach, and keep the following points in mind:

- Focus on emphasising the facts, and not necessarily repeating myths too often.
- Provide explicit warnings before mentioning a myth to audiences.
- Communicate simply, with easy-to-understand arguments and stories.
- Be mindful of cultural cognition.
- Fill in any mental gaps left by discrediting misinformation with alternative explanations for why the myth is wrong. Alternatively, explain why someone might spread misinformation using persuasive, but untrue claims.

Debunking III: Make facts sticky

One of the problems with trying to replace mental gaps left by false ideas is that misinformation does not need to rely on scientific facts. It can be groundlessly sensational and tap into our emotions without having to rely on genuine data. This is what can make misinformation particularly memorable and mentally sticky. It is also why urban legends spread so readily. Though urban legends are fictional stories that start as hoaxes or false rumours, they can have an element of believability to them. Such legends are often passed on when they spark emotional reactions in their hearers, including feelings of disgust or surprise.[48] The challenge such stickiness poses for debunking misinformation, whether an urban legend or counter-vaccination untruths, is that it must be replaced with equally captivating facts. In short, it is necessary to "fight sticky myths with even stickier facts."[49] This will improve the chance that valid scientific facts will replace debunked falsehoods.

To understand how to make facts stickier it is worth looking at observations made by Chip and Dan Heath. The Heath brothers are academics and the authors of the bestselling book *Made to Stick: Why Some Ideas Survive and Others Die*. This book tackles questions of why some ideas, including urban legends and conspiracy theories, are sticky while others are not. Dan and Chip explain that sticky ideas tend to be "understood and remembered, and have a lasting impact – they change your audience's opinions or behavior."[50] How then can vaccination facts be made as sticky as antivaccination myths? According to the Heath brothers, sticky ideas tend to have six traits, which are captured in the acronym SUCCES: *Simple, Unexpected, Concrete, Credible, Emotional*, and *Story*. The stickiness of facts can be improved by implementing these six characteristics in messages, and no "special expertise is needed to apply these principles."[51] Therefore, the good news is that anyone can use the SUCCES acronym as a checklist to improve vaccine fact stickiness. The more of these six properties vaccine facts have, the greater potential that they may stick with audiences.

i Simple

The first step to making an idea sticky is to keep its message simple. This coincides with the debunking advice of trying to express messages simply. However, it does not necessarily mean just "dumbing down" the facts with fewer, less complicated words.[52] Instead, making a message truly simple means focussing on the core of an idea, and "stripping an idea down to its most critical essence."[53] In order to make a vaccination fact sticky, for instance, it is necessary to "weed out superfluous and tangential elements," and communicate the most important, core idea in as few words as possible.[54] It is vital to resist giving too much data and evidence. Instead hold fast to a single central idea that can be quickly and easily explained. Chip and Dan Heath state, "People are tempted to tell you everything, with perfect accuracy, right up front, when they should be giving you just enough info to be useful, then a little more, then a little more."[55] Simplicity is a process of prioritising the most fundamental point of a message first, rather than giving every fact and figure at once to audiences.

Making an idea simple also means ensuring that it is compact. Being compact means that an idea communicates profound insights in just a few words. Prime examples of compactness include proverbs, such as "two wrongs don't make a right", or "measure twice, cut once."[56] Such proverbs communicate important ideas in dense forms. As the Heath brothers explain: "We know that sentences are better than paragraphs. Two bullet points are better than five. Easy words are better than hard words. It's a bandwidth issue: The more we reduce the amount of information in an idea, the stickier it will be."[57] When it comes to the Simple characteristic then, remember this basic equation: **Simple = Core + Compact**.

Unfortunately, the science and safety of vaccines are complicated subjects to communicate to audiences. As a result, pro-vaccine advocates can struggle to make vaccination messages brief and understandable. Studies have further indicated that antivaccine media tends to be easier to read and comprehend than are provaccination messages.[58] Provaccine information often uses more complicated language and longer sentences.[59] Consequently, pro-vaccine supporters must keep the Simple trait at the forefront of vaccine advocacy, ensuring that they are delivering brief, easy to understand content.

ii Unexpected

Chip and Dan Heath explain that "Unexpected ideas are more likely to stick because surprise makes us pay attention and think."[60] The "extra attention and thinking" that such surprise triggers "sears unexpected events into our memories." A surprising message "jolts us to attention," which then captures people's focus and sustains interest.[61] The Surprise characteristic of sticky messaging can be generated by communicating something that is counterintuitive and unanticipated. Unexpectedness may be actuated by a startling idea that appears to defy common sense, making it seem unpredictable and stand out. In fact, common sense "is the enemy of sticky messages," because, when "messages sound like common sense, they float gently in one ear and out the other."[62] So remember, the Unexpected trait is actually the opposite of common sense and predictability.[63] When some news or idea is surprising it can grab people's attention by sparking curiosity. "How do we get our audience to pay attention to our ideas, and how do we maintain their interest when we need time to get the ideas across?" ask the Heath brothers.[64] "We need to violate people's expectations."

Taken as a whole, the following equation outlines this facet of sticky ideas: **Unexpected = Counterintuitive + Unpredictable**. What is noteworthy about this trait is that scientific findings can often seem counterintuitive. Though this might initially seem problematic, the counterintuitive nature of scientific data may actually make related ideas sticky if they are communicated in interesting ways. Does a vaccine fact seem unpredictable or surprising? If so, communicators should not shy away from that reality, and instead can use it to foster the stickiness of unexpected science in a message. Another potentially surprising fact, for instance, is that those who are spreading vaccine misinformation can be earning funds from their efforts.[65] Antivaccine champions who circulate conspiracy theories about sinister schemes to profit from vaccines, may themselves be turning a profit through social media monetisation. As a result, there is in fact a remarkable manner of conspiracy that can lie behind the spread of vaccine conspiracy theories. This involves income being made by fabricating conspiracies and getting online attention with false, sensational stories.

iii Concrete

Concrete ideas differ from abstract ones. They relate to things that can be described and detected directly by the human senses, and they tend to be easier to recall and mentally sticky. On the other hand, abstract ideas are concepts that are not easily connected to the physical world around us. They are less likely to be understood by our senses because they do not have a physical existence, and they are not associated with the same objects or events for everyone. Examples of abstract ideas include such concepts as *freedom, justice, personality*, or *infinity*. These are complex intellectual notions, which may mean very different things to different people. As a result, new abstract ideas can be difficult to understand and remember, making them less sticky. According to Chip and Dan Heath, "V8 engine is concrete. 'High-performance' is abstract."[66]

With these distinctions in mind, a message can be made stickier by relating it to concrete ideas, including physical actions, places, and bodily sensations. These concrete ideas can help to create mental visualisations for audiences about specific activities or stimulate sensory images and feelings. The Heath brothers provide an example from cookbook instructions to clarify how concrete messaging can be more helpful than trying to communicate abstract ideas. "[M]aybe you've experienced the frustration of cooking from a recipe that was too abstract: 'Cook until the mixture reaches a hearty consistency.' Huh? Just tell me how many minutes to stir! Show me a picture of what it looks like!"[67] The concreteness of a picture or a clear description of what the mixture should look like would be much more effective than an abstract idea such as "hearty consistency." Likewise, scientific ideas can be made stickier if we relate them to concrete actions, the senses, and clear physical descriptions rather than abstract ideas. Overall, remember that **Concrete = Actions + Senses**.

iv Credible

Chapter 3 outlined how antivaccination media features Source Cues. Recall that these cues include displays of academic qualifications, expertise, or references to scientific data and empirical evidence. Persuasion research has identified that audiences can rely upon such markers of expertise and credibility to make decisions. By the same token, Chip and Dan Heath explain that credibility improves a message's stickiness. If you want people to believe a message, it is vital "to find a source of credibility to draw on."[68] As the Heath brothers summarise, "Sticky ideas have to carry their own credentials."[69] In addition to highlighting a source's professional expertise, as well as employing reliable authorities or celebrities to communicate messages, credibility can also be boosted by using statistics (see Chapter 3).[70] Importantly, opinions of what is credible might vary from community to community. Some faith groups, for instance, may consider religious qualifications to be more authoritative than medical or scientific credentials. Consequently, a religious leader's opinion on vaccines could be held in greater esteem than might medical and scientific credentials.[71]

Finally, trustworthiness and honesty further enhance credibility.[72] A message will likely be less sticky if it is perceived to be dishonest by audiences. By and large then, when trying to make vaccine messages stickier, remember that **Credible = Expertise + Honesty**. As I have maintained about government marketing of COVID-19 vaccines, such "messages must be honest and transparent above all. Distrust in government, pharmaceutical companies, as well as health systems can trigger vaccine hesitancy, and any hint of dishonesty may feed further suspicions."[73] Honesty should be a key attribute of all vaccine advocacy, which lends credibility to information in counter-vaccine misinformation-rich environments. On a similar note, the Credible trait of sticky communications also means that vaccination advocates should keep in mind how they too can harness Source Cues for themselves, including employing clear markers of expertise and consensus.

Improving credibility and consensus

During casual conversations with people expressing vaccine hesitancy, I find that it is not uncommon to be asked whether I have heard the latest vaccination news. Have I read a report that a particular vaccine has finally been proven unsafe, or about recent findings unveiling that government and pharmaceuticals have been found out for hiding the truth about vaccine dangers? When I am asked such questions, I have occasionally enquired about where the questioner first heard such astonishing details. Typically, I am told that the evidence was obtained from an online source, often passed on by a friend or family member who shared a social media link. At the same time, individuals assure me that the information is credible. It came from an expert, such as a rogue doctor or scientist who is trying to open the eyes of the public to the truth of vaccines.

What is fascinating about these exchanges is that analyses of counter-science media demonstrate that such communications put notable effort into establishing that they are credible.[74] As explained in Chapter 3, this includes references to the apparent expertise and supposed heaps of scientific evidence that support counter-science arguments and conspiracies. It is also the case that counter-science media can appeal to credibility far more frequently than pro-science communications usually do.[75] Counter-science media is regularly in the business of making itself look credible and appearing as though it is backed up by science while spreading false ideas. Social media's ability to distribute such seemingly credible disinformation is why it has been criticised by researchers.[76] Yet, it has also been recognised that "online media offer scientists more opportunities to communicate directly with the general public rather than having to rely on journalists as mediators."[77]

Therefore, we know that misinformation spreads online, and that it is often made to look like it is coming from credible sources. We also know that online media can be used to reach the public with pro-science messages. Research has further indicated that when online media that refutes misinformation comes from a credible and trustworthy source, such as the Centers for Disease Control, it is effective in reducing people's misperceptions.[78] In fact, when a source like the CDC corrects misinformation online, it can be "sufficiently persuasive that it affects everyone."[79] This highlights the power of credibility that truly reliable, expert sources may have, even amongst the noise of social media and online communications. As another study concluded about debunking autism myths, corrections "are more effective if they come from a person or institution that is high in perceived credibility." This perceived credibility is linked to the trustworthiness that such sources convey to audiences.

In keeping with the Credible principle of message stickiness, pro-vaccine communications should utilise Source Cues whenever possible (Chapter 3), because signals of expertise can be effective when refuting misinformation. If you are a researcher, a doctor, an allied health practitioner, then highlight your own credentials and your affiliations with reputable universities, research institutes, state health services and hospitals. Pro-vaccination messages will be more effective when they are associated with respectable organisations and trustworthy sources, and such genuine credibility must be clearly voiced. If you are not an expert, correct vaccine misinformation using resources from highly regarded sources, such as the Centers for Disease Control or comparable institutions. In relation to these suggestions, it can also be helpful to refer to scientific consensus, and the fact that the majority of scientific evidence supports the safety and efficacy of vaccines.

One study examined this strategy in relation to people's attitudes toward vaccines and the discredited autism–vaccine link. In the end, the authors found that it can be effective to communicate to audiences that "a preponderance of scientific evidence refutes a link [between autism and vaccines] and that scientists overwhelming agree than none exists."[80] Similarly, another study has observed that telling people "90 percent of medical scientists agree that vaccines are safe and that all parents should be required to vaccinate their children" significantly reduced people's anxieties about vaccines and belief in an autism–vaccine relationship.[81] The researchers concluded that emphasising "medical consensus increases perceived scientific agreement," and this acts as a sort of "'gateway' belief by promoting favorable public attitudes toward vaccination as well as by reducing perceived risk and belief in the (long discredited) autism–vaccine link."[82] Publicising the scientific consensus on vaccines is important. This is the case not only because such consensus is convincing, but also because it is an honest representation of the scientific landscape. The empirical data, arguments, and academic agreement are solidly in support of vaccines, and it can be valuable to inform people about that actuality.

A communicator's perceived credibility can also be strengthened through the quality of evidence that a messenger provides. This has been described as "intrinsic credibility," and it is based on the strength of the arguments a communication puts forward, which are anchored to the message's factual proofs.[83] This intrinsic credibility is contrasted with the "extrinsic credibility" stemming from an individual's qualifications and outward markers of expertise. As one study concluded, "Effective health messages need to be well grounded in information that is immediately seen as sound," which serves to enhance the communication's credibility.[84] The good news about intrinsic credibility is that the quality of evidence for vaccine safety and effectiveness rests squarely on the side of vaccination. Even if you do not have the degrees or institutional associations meriting extrinsic credibility, there is a surplus of factual evidence and quality sources that can be used to ensure intrinsic credibility for pro-vaccine messages.

When considering the Credible element of message stickiness, it is important to keep in mind that antivaccination media regularly packages misinformation as though it comes from an expert, reliable source. In many ways, that makes it particularly vital for pro-vaccine advocacy to be clearly identified as coming from truly reputable sources as well. It should demonstrate that it originates from actual experts who agree in consensus, and is supported by a substantial majority of scientific evidence.

v Emotional

In Chapter 4 it was explained that references to vaccine risks and dangers often form the backbone of antivaccination messages. The influence of such claims is tied to the persuasive cue described as the Arousal of Fear. People are also more likely to share communications that they find worrying. Though fear is not the only emotion that is attention-grabbing, including some emotional component to a communication can increase its stickiness. "How do we get people to care about our ideas?" ask Chip and Dan Heath.[85] "We make them *feel* something." For the Heath brothers, employing emotions is "not about pushing people's emotional buttons."[86] Instead, the "goal of making messages 'emotional' is to make people care," because, "Feelings inspire people to act."[87] As they make clear, "Belief counts for a lot, but belief isn't enough. For people to take action, they have to *care*."[88]

Caring about people and beliefs is tied to the emotions that they elicit. This is why emotions play such a central role in helping certain ideas to stick and spread. If individuals care about certain ideas, they are far more likely to pass on and defend them. Chip and Dan Heath further explain that it can be beneficial to focus a message's emotions upon an audience's self-interest, which improves its mental adhesiveness. Inform an audience, for instance, exactly what benefits an idea will gain them, since it "will come as no surprise that one reliable way of making people care is by invoking self-interest."[89] This can be enhanced by frequently using the word "you," which can make a message hit home emotionally.[90] For example, rather than stating that vaccines can give *people* a feeling of health security, note that vaccines can give *you* a feeling of safety. Communicators should also be cautious about trying to activate negative emotions in audiences, because trying to shame or frighten can be counterproductive.[91] Rather than using fear to get people to care, consider trying to kindle positive emotions, including feelings of hope, happiness, and empathy.

To simplify: **Emotional = Making People Care**. Additionally, when thinking about emotions, it is also helpful to consider the Moral Foundations Theory (Chapter 2). Remember that according to this theory, people can often make decisions in relation to emotionally driven moral intuitions. These emotional intuitions include the six central foundations of care/harm, fairness/cheating, loyalty/betrayal, authority/subversion, sanctity/degradation, and liberty/oppression.[92] Appeals to these moral foundations may improve the Emotional attribute and make vaccination facts stickier for audiences.

vi Stories

Chip and Dan Heath state that a key to making an idea sticky is to communicate the concept in the form of a story. Stories are effective because they can encourage audiences to roleplay and rehearse in their minds the ideas being communicated within a narrative. In a sense, a story acts as a sort of cerebral simulation, which can draw people in and invite them to experience ideas through their imaginations. Stories can also inspire people to action in ways that mere data often does not. As the Heath brothers conclude, "The story's power, then, is twofold: It provides simulation (knowledge about how to act) and inspiration (motivation to act)."[93]

As was made clear in Chapter 5, telling stories can often be far more persuasive than communicating sets of data or even trying to make well-reasoned arguments.[94] As a result, numerous researchers have advised that vaccine advocates use storytelling-based communications, because narratives are generally perceived by audiences to be less threatening than are attempts at logical argumentation.[95] Stories also seem to transcend people's education levels as they stimulate emotional reactions. Storytelling can also cultivate empathy, because people tend to personally identify with a storyline's characters, its contexts, as well as the values that a story is trying to communicate.[96] Indeed, storytelling is powerful, and put plainly: **Stories = Simulation + Inspiration**.

Sticky SUCCES

There is no sure-fire way to ensure that pro-science advocacy gets results. Not every individual will respond to intervention efforts in the same ways.

It can be difficult to forecast which types of messages, media posts, or in-person approaches will end up being sticky, and what ideas will go viral while others fade away. A further complicating factor is that the vaccine communications landscape is already littered with counter-vaccine messages that are often permeated with persuasive cues. As the Heath brothers have conceded, "It's hard to make ideas stick in a noisy, unpredictable, chaotic environment."[97] The vaccine advocacy environment is undoubtedly an unruly one. However, there are practical ways of improving communication efforts and making pro-vaccine messages stickier. To that end, it is of value to consider how the SUCCES principles can be used to improve vaccine advocacy.

Overview: How to Improve Vaccine Advocacy

After taking a deep dive into vaccine advocacy techniques, ranging from general guidelines to making facts stickier, what results is a substantial amount of information to absorb. In a bid to simplify this vast breadth of material, the following summary highlights crucial advice to remember.

I Initial Suggestions

Vaccine advocacy can be improved by starting with these seven recommendations:

i Discard the Information Deficit Model

Counterintuitively, research has found that increasing people's factual knowledge about vaccines often does not translate into vaccine confidence or improved vaccination behaviours. In fact, just trying to correct vaccine misinformation with scientific facts can occasionally be disadvantageous. People have a tendency to support whatever vaccination position aligns best with the core values maintained in their social groups, rather than simply making decisions based upon objective facts.

ii Target fence-sitters

Focus on reaching vaccine hesitant fence-sitters, who may have uncertainties and doubts, but who are not ardent vaccine deniers. Fence-sitters represent a much larger segment of the public, and they will be far more amenable to vaccine advocacy.

iii Tailor messages

Adapt messages for the audiences you are hoping to reach. Take into account the informational needs, cultural contexts, social values, and worries expressed by those towards whom vaccine advocacy is aimed. Also consider employing tailored cultural-identity affirmation or pluralistic advocacy to help alleviate negative identity-protective cognition reactions.

iv Be respectful, empathetic and audience-focussed

Dedicating time to listen to vaccine hesitant individuals and treating people with dignity is essential. It may be tempting to dismiss people's vaccine doubts outright, while it can also be challenging to make time to thoughtfully respond to vaccine questions. Nevertheless, respectfully listening to someone's concerns, and keeping dialogue open, can play a key role in people's vaccine decision-making processes. It also increases trust. Keep in mind that Motivational Interviewing is one of the few intervention strategies with positive results. Additionally, a method of improving your listening aptitudes for MI is the HURIER model.

v Avoid verbal aggression

Even though antivaccination messages are factually untrue, and you may feel very strongly about vaccines, it is important to refrain from being hostile. Aggressive language is polarising, and people react negatively to being ridiculed or treated as unintelligent. Verbal aggression decreases an individual's perceptions of your credibility and likeability, and it reduces an audience's motivation to learn.

vi Be honest and open to questions

It is necessary to be open to questions and honest about facts. Not being open to questions fuels pre-existing scepticism and distrust. Being honest means communicating both the potential side effects of vaccines, as well as the possible health effects caused by vaccine-preventable diseases.

vii Acknowledge people's fears

Dismissing people's vaccine fears can fuel distrust. Such fears stem from genuine concerns for the wellbeing of loved ones. Brushing off people's safety concerns can be perceived as devaluing people's gut feelings about trying to safeguard the people who they love.

II Additional Techniques

There are several intervention strategies that can improve confidence in vaccines and increase vaccine uptake. These include behaviour-modification techniques, such as removing access barriers, applying incentives and penalties, as well as nudging (Chapter 5). Yet in the end, recommendations from doctors, nurses, and pharmacists remain one of the most influential factors in people's vaccine decision-making processes. The following approaches can be used by healthcare workers and members of the general public to improve interactions with hesitant individuals

i Make presumptive announcements

Vaccine acceptance increases when the option of getting vaccinated is framed in the form of a presumptive announcement. For example, "Let's book an appointment now for the vaccinations your child needs."

ii Emphasise social consensus, norms, and the common good

Many people choose to get vaccinated because they believe, correctly, that most other people are doing so. Emphasising that the majority of people get vaccinated can accompany a presumptive announcement: "This vaccine is accepted by the majority of people attending this practice." It also highlights how vaccination is the social norm and the assumed default action for all patients. It can also be helpful to point out that vaccines serve the common good.

iii Ask self-predictive questions

Inviting individuals to consider their future intentions to vaccinate, such as by asking people to formulate date-specific plans, may improve the likelihood that they will follow through with that intention later.

iv Tell stories

Stories can be more persuasive than logical, fact-centred arguments. Telling personal narratives about how you or others became convinced of vaccine safety and effectiveness, or why you chose to vaccinate yourself or others, can be more engaging and influential.

v Affirm autonomy of choice

Support people's personal autonomy and emphasise that in the end individuals have the freedom to make important immunisation decisions. Verbally affirming personal autonomy can alleviate feelings of being forced into vaccinating. It can also open up room for further conversations, and is a means of empowering people. Hesitant individuals should be asked whether they would like more information about vaccines to make their own informed decisions.

III Debunking and pre-bunking

Refuting vaccine misinformation is a difficult but much needed task. Debunking vaccination myths more effectively, and inoculating audiences against misinformation can assist in the cause.

i Truth sandwich

When debunking a vaccine myth, try using the truth sandwich Fact–Myth–Fallacy–Fact structure: 1. Fact: State the truth first; 2: Myth: Warn that misinformation is false and state a myth only once; 3. Fallacy: Explain why the misinformation is wrong and what tricks are being used to promote it; 4. Fact: Affirm the genuine facts again.

ii Pre-bunking

Exposing the tricks in vaccine misinformation will make individuals better at recognising false claims and persuasion tactics in the future. This can mentally inoculate people against myths. Research suggests that pre-bunking is more effective than trying to debunk after misinformation has already been accepted.

IV Sticky facts

Facts can be made catchier by using the SUCCES model for making information sticky.

i   Simple: Communicate the core idea compactly, using as few words as possible, and ensure that it is easy to understand for non-experts. **Simple = Core + Compact**.

ii Unexpected: Stress how a fact is surprising to catch people's attention. How does it go against common sense or how is it unpredictable? **Unexpected = Counterintuitive + Unpredictable**.

iii Concrete: Connect facts to physical actions, specific places, and the senses, which can stimulate sensory images, mental visuals, and feelings. **Concreteness = Actions + Senses**.

iv Credible: Highlight expertise through academic qualifications, professional experience, or references to scientific data and empirical evidence. Honesty improves credibility, and it is beneficial to emphasise scientific consensus. **Credible = Expertise + Honesty**.

v   Emotional: Try to kindle positive emotions, including feelings of hope, happiness, and empathy. Emotions cause people to care about facts. **Emotional = Making People Care**.

vi Story: Increase stickiness by communicating ideas in the form of a story. Stories are memorable, they inspire, and they help people simulate situations in their minds. **Stories = Simulation + Inspiration**.

A call to action

The advice collated above reflects many successes and failures researchers from around the world have observed when trying to lessen vaccine hesitancy. The substance of these recommendations is rooted in an assortment of studies and theories from a variety of fields that have been outlined throughout this book's chapters. These chapters have also examined the science, safety, and effectiveness of vaccines, as well as the historical foundations of modern vaccine-scepticism. The primary reasons why some people are vaccine hesitant have also been discussed, from distrust to sociocultural beliefs, values to risk calculations, social networks and online media. The book further consolidates practical insights about the psychology lying behind why people have vaccine worries, and the key factors that influence vaccine decision-making. Leading vaccine myths have been explained, including conspiratorial notions that BigPharma and health authorities are covering up vaccine dangers in pursuit of profit. The persuasive cues scattered throughout antivaccination arguments were also decoded, including appeals to credibility, social proof, and underdog effects. Altogether, this has provided empirically grounded advice on the most effective ways of responding to vaccine hesitant individuals.

Having now covered this expanse of information, I thought that I would conclude with a personal story of my own. I am a proud dad of two adopted kids. In fact, I have frequently told my boys that if the only thing I ever truly accomplished in life was adopting them, and being a dedicated father, then the meaning of my life has been already fulfilled. The elder son had a medical history that included repeated bouts of pneumonia before we adopted him. The first months of his life were marked with monthly cases requiring repeated medical intervention. Then, after we adopted him, he once again came down with a severe case of pneumonia.

If you are a parent, you may be familiar with the special variety of suffering reserved for moms and dads who have to watch their kids in pain. In fact, that is one of the reasons why parents are hesitant about having their own children vaccinated. They recoil from the idea of putting their kids in distress and discomfort. This, even though getting vaccinated may result in a short span flash of pain, which will conceivably keep children from much worse physical anguish over the course of their lives. Nevertheless, it was remarkably difficult to watch my son struggle to breath and hear him scream when we had to leave him on his own in the radiology room so that his chest could be x-rayed. He healed up from that episode, but after we moved from Canada to Australia, my son once again came down with pneumonia symptoms. Our family doctor, who was also a teaching physician at the University of Queensland, investigated our son's medical records. In doing so, our GP suggested that he receive an additional booster dose of the 13vPCV pneumococcal conjugate vaccine, because the extra booster is recommended for at-risk children in Australia. Plus, there was some doubt about our son's pre-adoption vaccine records. We readily agreed with the medical advice, and our son received the booster dose.

The years have gone by, and my son has never again experienced a single case of pneumonia. Interestingly, it was only after several pneumonia-free years that we thought back to that booster shot, and the fact that from then on, a child who had experienced monthly bouts of pneumonia ceased having any more incidents of it. That is an example of both the power of vaccination as well as why vaccines can be a victim of their own success. Once people get vaccinated, they can cease to notice the truly significant impact that they have, since vaccines prevent illnesses from occurring in the first place. We also can have short memories regarding diseases such as smallpox, polio, diphtheria, and even pneumonia, which devastated lives before vaccines helped keep them in check throughout many regions of the world. As for myself, I had never truly witnessed the effects of polio until I travelled abroad as young adult. It was only then that I considered the importance of polio vaccines, after I saw the repercussions of vaccine preventable diseases with my own eyes. At the same time, it was easy to forget my own son's medical history after a vaccine prevented him from developing pneumonia again. We also tend to forget that even if we personally do not feel at risk from certain diseases, getting ourselves vaccinated helps to protect those who are more vulnerable.

Even so, I became a vaccine advocate not solely because of these experiences. I have also never received any funds or profited from associations with pharmaceutical companies. Instead, the primary reason why I actively support vaccines is down to years spent examining the impact of vaccination, vaccine safety, and vaccine effectiveness in academic peer-reviewed research. This has coincided with my academic career, which has been devoted to studying counter-science misinformation and media persuasion. The global impacts of such science-skepticism, in contrast with the empirical evidence supporting the safety and effectiveness of vaccines, troubled me enough to act. With that said, I would like to end this book by asking you, the reader, to also take action. Are there ways that you can apply various ideas and advice offered throughout this book to support vaccination in your own local or online contexts? Do you have your own positive vaccine story to share with your community? Perhaps you can think of new methods of improving vaccine advocacy. There are likely creative approaches for reducing vaccine hesitancy that no one has yet thought of. You may be able to unearth such novel approaches for the first time. The expectation, therefore, is that this book is not merely a source of helpful information but also possibly serves as a pre-bunking exercise. It is further hoped that it is a call to action. One that sparks an interest in advocating for vaccination in better ways, through a richer understanding of vaccines, vaccine hesitancy, and antivaccination.

Notes

1 Jim Underdown, "The Salton Sea Flat Earth Test: When Skeptics Meet Deniers," *Skeptical Inquirer*, https://skepticalinquirer.org/2018/11/the-salton-sea-flat-earth-test-when-skeptics-meet-deniers/; Ross Blocher, "Salton Sea Earth

Curvature Test," Center for Inquiry, https://cfiig.org/earth-curvature-test/; CFI, "When Skeptics Meet Deniers – CFI Investigations Group Tests Flat Earth Claims," Center for Inquiry Investigations Group https://www.youtube.com/watch?v=CnrjdD08dWg.

2 Julie Leask, "Target the Fence-Sitters," *Nature* 473, no. 7348 (2011).

3 Philipp Schmid et al., "How to Respond to Vocal Vaccine Deniers in Public," *Vaccine* 36, no. 2 (2016): 196.

4 Julie Leask, "Should We Do Battle with Antivaccination Activists?," *Public Health Research & Practice* 25, no. 2 (2015): 3.

5 Ibid.

6 Mia Liza A. Lustria et al., "A Meta-Analysis of Web-Delivered Tailored Health Behavior Change Interventions," *Journal of Health Communication* 18, no. 9 (2013); Charitha Gowda et al., "A Pilot Study on the Effects of Individually Tailored Education for MMR Vaccine-Hesitant Parents on MMR Vaccination Intention," *Human Vaccines & Immunotherapeutics* 9, no. 2 (2013); Robb Butler and Noni E. Macdonald, "Diagnosing the Determinants of Vaccine Hesitancy in Specific Subgroups: The Guide to Tailoring Immunization Programmes (TIP)," *Vaccine* 33, no. 34 (2015); Suellen Hopfer, "Effects of a Narrative HPV Vaccination Intervention Aimed at Reaching College Women: A Randomized Controlled Trial," *Prevention Science* 13, no. 2 (2012); Mary A. Gerend, Melissa A. Shepherd, and Mia Liza A. Lustria, "Increasing Human Papillomavirus Vaccine Acceptability by Tailoring Messages to Young Adult Women's Perceived Barriers," *Sexually Transmitted Diseases* 40, no. 5 (2013).

7 Robert John and Marshall K. Cheney, "Resistance to Influenza Vaccination: Psychographics, Audience Segments, and Potential Promotions to Increase Vaccination," *Social Marketing Quarterly* 14, no. 2 (2008).

8 Gabrielle M. Bryden et al., "Anti-Vaccination and Pro-Cam Attitudes Both Reflect Magical Beliefs About Health," *Vaccine* 36, no. 9 (2018); Lesley Gray et al., "Community Responses to Communication Campaigns for Influenza a (H1N1): A Focus Group Study," *BMC Public Health* 12, no. 1 (2012).

9 Lustria et al., "A Meta-Analysis of Web-Delivered Tailored Health Behavior Change Interventions," 1040.

10 Ibid.

11 B. Nyhan et al., "Effective Messages in Vaccine Promotion: A Randomized Trial," *Pediatrics* 133, no. 4 (2014).

12 Ibid., 838.

13 Ibid., 839.

14 Man-pui Sally Chan et al., "Debunking: A Meta-Analysis of the Psychological Efficacy of Messages Countering Misinformation," *Psychological Science* 28, no. 11 (2017); Ullrich Ecker, Stephan Lewandowsky, and David Tang, "Explicit Warnings Reduce but Do Not Eliminate the Continued Influence of Misinformation," *Memory & Cognition* 38, no. 8 (2010); Stephan Lewandowsky et al., "Misinformation and Its Correction," *Psychological Science in the Public Interest* 13, no. 3 (2012).

15 Sara Pluviano, Caroline Watt, and Sergio Della Sala, "Misinformation Lingers in Memory: Failure of Three Pro-Vaccination Strategies," *PLoS One* 12, no. 7 (2017): 1.

16 John Cook and Stephan Lewandowsky, *The Debunking Handbook* (St Lucia: University of Queensland, 2011); Stephan Lewandowsky et al., *The Debunking Handbook* (Fairfax: George Mason University, 2020).

17 Cook and Lewandowsky, *The Debunking Handbook*, 2.

18 Lewandowsky et al., "Misinformation and Its Correction."

19 Ethan Porter and Thomas J. Wood, *False Alarm: The Truth About Political Mistruths in the Trump Era* (Cambridge: Cambridge University Press, 2019); Briony

Swire-Thompson, Joseph DeGutis, and David Lazer, "Searching for the Backfire Effect: Measurement and Design Considerations," *Journal of Applied Research in Memory and Cognition* 9, no. 3 (2020); Thomas Wood and Ethan Porter, "The Elusive Backfire Effect: Mass Attitudes' Steadfast Factual Adherence," *Political Behavior* 41, no. 1 (2018).

20 Lewandowsky et al., *The Debunking Handbook*, 9.

21 Ibid., 13.

22 Ullrich Ecker, Joshua Hogan, and Stephan Lewandowsky, "Reminders and Repetition of Misinformation: Helping or Hindering Its Retraction?," *Journal of Applied Research in Memory and Cognition* 6, no. 2 (2017).

23 Floyd H. Allport and Milton Lepkin, "Wartime Rumors of Waste and Special Privilege: Why Some People Believe Them," *The Journal of Abnormal and Social Psychology* 40, no. 1 (1945).

24 Lawrence E. Boehm, "The Validity Effect: A Search for Mediating Variables," *Personality and Social Psychology Bulletin* 20, no. 3 (1994): 285.

25 Ibid.

26 Anne L. Roggeveen and Gita Venkataramani Johar, "Perceived Source Variability Versus Familiarity: Testing Competing Explanations for the Truth Effect," *Journal of Consumer Psychology* 12, no. 2 (2002): 81.

27 Lewandowsky et al., *The Debunking Handbook*, 15.

28 Cook and Lewandowsky, *The Debunking Handbook*, 2.

29 Lewandowsky et al., *The Debunking Handbook*, 11–13; Laura M König, "Debunking Nutrition Myths: An Experimental Test of the 'Truth Sandwich' Text Format," *PsyArXiv Preprints* (2022); Margaret Sullivan, "Instead of Trump's Propaganda, How About a Nice 'Truth Sandwich'?," *The Washington Post*, https://www.washingtonpost.com/lifestyle/style/instead-of-trumps-propaganda-how-about-a-nice-truth-sandwich/2018/06/15/80df8c36-70af-11e8-bf86-a2351b5ece99_story.html; Sean Illing, "How the Media Should Respond to Trump's Lies: State of the Union Edition," *Vox*, https://www.vox.com/2018/11/15/18047360/trump-state-of-the-union-speech-2019-george-lakoff.

30 Eric Bonetto et al., "Priming Resistance to Persuasion Decreases Adherence to Conspiracy Theories," *Social Influence* 13, no. 3 (2018): 126.

31 Daniel Jolley and Karen M. Douglas, "Prevention Is Better Than Cure: Addressing Anti-Vaccine Conspiracy Theories," *Journal of Applied Social Psychology* 47, no. 8 (2017): 466.

32 Ibid., 465.

33 Ibid., 467.

34 Lewandowsky et al., *The Debunking Handbook*, 7; Cook and Lewandowsky, *The Debunking Handbook*, 5.

35 Lewandowsky et al., "Misinformation and Its Correction"; Ecker, Lewandowsky, and Tang, "Explicit Warnings Reduce but Do Not Eliminate the Continued Influence of Misinformation."

36 Jolley and Douglas, "Prevention Is Better Than Cure: Addressing Anti-Vaccine Conspiracy Theories," 467.

37 Cook and Lewandowsky, *The Debunking Handbook*, 3.

38 Muhammad Amith et al., "Using Pathfinder Networks to Discover Alignment between Expert and Consumer Conceptual Knowledge from Online Vaccine Content," *Journal of Biomedical Informatics* 74 (2017); Catalina L. Toma and Jonathan D. D'Angelo, "Tell-Tale Words: Linguistic Cues Used to Infer the Expertise of Online Medical Advice," *Journal of Language and Social Psychology* 34, no. 1 (2015).

39 Tsuyoshi Okuhara et al., "A Readability Comparison of Anti- Versus Pro-Influenza Vaccination Online Messages in Japan," *Preventive Medicine Reports* 6 (2017).

40 Cook and Lewandowsky, *The Debunking Handbook*, 3.
41 Ibid.
42 Lewandowsky et al., *The Debunking Handbook*, 11.
43 Dan Kahan, "Fixing the Communications Failure," *Nature* 463, no. 7279 (2010): 297; "Cultural Cognition as a Conception of the Cultural Theory of Risk," in *Handbook of Risk Theory: Epistemology, Decision Theory, Ethics, and Social Implications of Risk*, ed. Sabine Roeser, et al. (Dordrecht: Springer, 2012), 752–53.
44 Lewandowsky et al., *The Debunking Handbook*, 12.
45 Cook and Lewandowsky, *The Debunking Handbook*, 5.
46 John Cook, "Busting Myths: A Practical Guide to Countering Science Denial," *The Conversation*, https://theconversation.com/busting-myths-a-practical-guide-to-countering-science-denial-42618.
47 Chan et al., "Debunking: A Meta-Analysis of the Psychological Efficacy of Messages Countering Misinformation."; Ecker, Lewandowsky, and Tang, "Explicit Warnings Reduce but Do Not Eliminate the Continued Influence of Misinformation"; Lewandowsky et al., "Misinformation and Its Correction."
48 Chip Heath, Chris Bell, and Emily Sternberg, "Emotional Selection in Memes: The Case of Urban Legends," *Journal of Personality and Social Psychology* 81, no. 6 (2001).
49 Cook, "Busting Myths: A Practical Guide to Countering Science Denial".
50 Chip Heath and Dan Heath, *Made to Stick: Why Some Ideas Survive and Others Die*, 1st ed. (New York: Random House, 2007), 8.
51 Ibid., 18.
52 Ibid., 27.
53 Ibid., 28.
54 Ibid.
55 Ibid., 57.
56 Ibid., 47.
57 Ibid., 45.
58 Okuhara et al., "A Readability Comparison of Anti- Versus Pro-Influenza Vaccination Online Messages in Japan."
59 Anna Kata, "A Postmodern Pandora's Box: Anti-Vaccination Misinformation on the Internet," *Vaccine* 28, no. 7 (2010): 36–41; Gabriele Sak et al., "Comparing the Quality of Pro- and Anti-Vaccination Online Information: A Content Analysis of Vaccination-Related Webpages," *BMC Public Health* 16, no. 1 (2016): 9.
60 Heath and Heath, *Made to Stick: Why Some Ideas Survive and Others Die*, 68.
61 Ibid., 67.
62 Ibid., 72.
63 Ibid., 71.
64 Ibid., 16.
65 Aliaksandr Herasimenka et al., "The Political Economy of Digital Profiteering: Communication Resource Mobilization by Anti-Vaccination Actors," *Journal of Communication* (2022).
66 Heath and Heath, *Made to Stick: Why Some Ideas Survive and Others Die*, 104.
67 Ibid., 106.
68 Ibid., 163.
69 Ibid., 17.
70 Ibid., 141.
71 Retna Siwi Padmawati et al., "Religious and Community Leaders' Acceptance of Rotavirus Vaccine Introduction in Yogyakarta, Indonesia: A Qualitative Study," *BMC Public Health* 19, no. 1 (2019); Harapan Harapan et al., "Religion

and Measles Vaccination in Indonesia, 1991–2017," *American Journal of Preventive Medicine* 60, no. 1 (2021).

72 Heath and Heath, *Made to Stick: Why Some Ideas Survive and Others Die*, 137.

73 Tom Aechtner, "Vaccine Deniers Are a Minority in Australia but a Successful Rollout Hinges on Facts and Honesty," *The Guardian*, https://www.theguardia n.com/commentisfree/2021/jan/14/vaccine-deniers-are-a-minority-in-australia -but-a-successful-rollout-hinges-on-facts-and-honesty.

74 Thomas Aechtner, "Online in the Evolution Wars: An Analysis of Young Earth Creationism Cyber-Propaganda," *The Australian Religious Studies Review* 23, no. 3 (2010); Aechtner, "Darwin-Skeptic Mass Media: Examining Persuasion in the Evolution Wars," *Journal of Media and Religion* 13, no. 4 (2014); Aechtner, "Distrust, Danger, and Confidence: A Content Analysis of the Australian Vac- cination-Risks Network Blog," *Public Understanding of Science* (2020); Aechtner, "Improving Evolution Advocacy: Translating Vaccine Interventions to the Evolution Wars," *Zygon* 55, no. 1 (2020).

75 Thomas Aechtner, "Challenging the Darwin-Skeptics: Examining Proevolu- tionist Media Persuasion," *Journal of Media and Religion* 15, no. 2 (2016); Aechtner, *Media and Science-Religion Conflict: Mass Persuasion in the Evolution Wars* (Abingdon, Oxon: Routledge, 2020).

76 Lewandowsky Stephan et al., "Misinformation and Its Correction: Continued Influence and Successful Debiasing," *Psychological Science in the Public Interest* 13, no. 3 (2012); Alessandro Bessi et al., "Science vs Conspiracy: Collective Narra- tives in the Age of Misinformation," *PLoS One* 10, no. 2 (2015).

77 Hans Peter Peters et al., "Public Communication of Science 2.0: Is the Com- munication of Science Via the 'New Media' Online a Genuine Transformation or Old Wine in New Bottles?," *EMBO Rep* 15, no. 7 (2014).

78 Emily K. Vraga and Leticia Bode, "Using Expert Sources to Correct Health Misinformation in Social Media," *Science Communication* 39, no. 5 (2017).

79 Ibid., 635.

80 Christopher E. Clarke et al., "The Influence of Weight-of-Evidence Messages on (Vaccine) Attitudes: A Sequential Mediation Model," *Journal of Health Com- munication* 20, no. 11 (2015): 1306.

81 Sander L. van der Linden, Chris E. Clarke, and Edward W. Maibach, "High- lighting Consensus among Medical Scientists Increases Public Support for Vac- cines: Evidence from a Randomized Experiment," *BMC Public Health* 15, no. 1207 (2015): 1.

82 Ibid., 3.

83 Dale Hample and Jessica M. Hample, "Persuasion About Health Risks: Evi- dence, Credibility, Scientific Flourishes, and Risk Perceptions," *Argumentation and Advocacy* 51, no. 1 (2014): 17.

84 Ibid., 27.

85 Heath and Heath, *Made to Stick: Why Some Ideas Survive and Others Die*, 17.

86 Ibid., 168.

87 Ibid., 169.

88 Ibid., 168.

89 Ibid., 177.

90 Ibid., 181.

91 Joshua Greenberg, Eve Dubé, and Michelle Driedger, "Vaccine Hesitancy: In Search of the Risk Communication Comfort Zone," *PLoS Currents* 9 (2017).

92 Jonathan Haidt and Jesse Graham, "When Morality Opposes Justice: Con- servatives Have Moral Intuitions That Liberals May Not Recognize," *Social Jus- tice Research* 20, no. 1 (2007): 104–06.

93 Heath and Heath, *Made to Stick: Why Some Ideas Survive and Others Die*, 206.

94 Anna Winterbottom et al., "Does Narrative Information Bias Individual's Decision Making? A Systematic Review," *Social Science & Medicine* 67, no. 12 (2008); Rachel M. Cunningham and Julie A. Boom, "Telling Stories of Vaccine-Preventable Diseases: Why It Works," *South Dakota Medicine* (2013); Adebanke L. Adebayo et al., "The Effectiveness of Narrative Versus Didactic Information Formats on Pregnant Women's Knowledge, Risk Perception, Self-Efficacy, and Information Seeking Related to Climate Change Health Risks," *International Journal of Environmental Research and Public Health* 17, no. 19 (2020); Chingching Chang, "Increasing Mental Health Literacy Via Narrative Advertising," *Journal of Health Communication* 13, no. 1 (2008); Sheila T. Murphy et al., "Comparing the Relative Efficacy of Narrative vs Nonnarrative Health Messages in Reducing Health Disparities Using a Randomized Trial," *American Journal of Public Health* 105, no. 10 (2015).

95 Hopfer, "Effects of a Narrative HPV Vaccination Intervention Aimed at Reaching College Women: A Randomized Controlled Trial."

96 Kenneth Holler and Anthony Scalzo, "'I've Heard Some Things That Scare Me'. Responding with Empathy to Parents' Fears of Vaccinations," *Missouri Medicine* 109, no. 1 (2012); Luz Martínez Martínez et al., "Formulas for Prevention, Narrative Versus Non-Narrative Formats. A Comparative Analysis of Their Effects on Young People's Knowledge, Attitude and Behaviour in Relation to HPV," *Revista Latina de Comunicación Social*, no. 73 (2018); Ubaldo Cuesta, Luz Martínez, and Victoria Cuesta, "Effectiveness of Narrative Persuasion on Facebook: Change of Attitude and Intention Towards HPV," *European Journal of Social Science Education and Research* 4, no. 6 (2017).

97 Heath and Heath, *Made to Stick: Why Some Ideas Survive and Others Die*, 27.

Index

Printed in the United States
by Baker & Taylor Publisher Services